The Challenges of Creating a Global Health Resource Tracking System

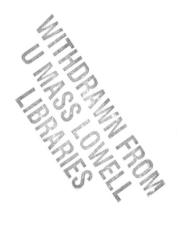

Elisa Eiseman, Donna Fossum

Sponsored by the Bill & Melinda Gates Foundation

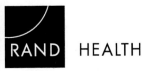

HEALTH

This research was sponsored by the Global Health Policy Research Network, a program of the Center for Global Development, sponsored by the Bill & Melinda Gates Foundation and conducted by RAND Health, a division of the RAND Corporation.

Library of Congress Cataloging-in-Publication Data

Eiseman, Elisa.
    The challenges of creating a global health resource tracking system / Elisa Eiseman, Donna Fossum.
      p. cm.
    "MG-317."
    Includes bibliographical references.
    ISBN 0-8330-3727-7 (pbk. : alk. paper)
    1. World health. 2. Health care rationing. 3. Public health surveillance. 4. Public health—Research—Methodology. 5. Public health—International cooperation.
    [DNLM: 1. Health Care Rationing. 2. World Health. 3. Data Collection. 4. Health Resources—organization & administration. 5. Health Resources—statistics & numerical data. 6. International Cooperation.] I. Fossum, Donna, 1949– II.Title.

RA441.E375 2005
362.1'072—dc22

The RAND Corporation is a nonprofit research organization providing objective analysis and effective solutions that address the challenges facing the public and private sectors around the world. RAND's publications do not necessarily reflect the opinions of its research clients and sponsors.

RAND® is a registered trademark.

Published 2005 by the RAND Corporation
1776 Main Street, P.O. Box 2138, Santa Monica, CA 90407-2138
1200 South Hayes Street, Arlington, VA 22202-5050
201 North Craig Street, Suite 202, Pittsburgh, PA 15213-1516
RAND URL: http://www.rand.org/
To order RAND documents or to obtain additional information, contact
Distribution Services: Telephone: (310) 451-7002;
Fax: (310) 451-6915; Email: order@rand.org

Preface

Developed countries, international organizations, and other entities provide substantial amounts of aid each year to improve the health of people in developing countries. These efforts are conducted by many entities across many activities at varying levels of scale. Currently, these health resource flows are not fully understood, and no information source exists to provide a "big picture" of who is giving what resources to whom and for what purpose. As a result, neither policymakers nor donors have the information they need to target these health resources as effectively as possible.

Would global efforts to improve health in developing countries be improved by a better and more comprehensive system for tracking health resources? If so, what data should such a global information source contain and how should the source be designed and used? As the first step in answering these questions, the RAND Corporation assessed the current state of global health resource tracking. This assessment asked the following: (1) What are the purposes and contents of existing health resource tracking systems that focus on developing countries? (2) What are the strengths and limitations of these systems? (3) What characteristics must a truly global health resource tracking system have in order to meet the needs of potential users and to address the limitations of current systems?

This report, which presents the results of the RAND assessment, contributes to answering these three and other relevant questions. The information presented was obtained through a series of extensive interviews with the key people involved in operating and/or managing all current major health resource data collections, as well as through detailed analyses of these data collections and reviews of literature. In addition, experts involved in health resource tracking were consulted at a gathering held at the RAND Corporation in May 2004. The intended audience for this report comprises policymakers and experts in international, national, and nongovernmental organizations, including both donor and recipient entities.

This research was sponsored by the Global Health Policy Research Network, a program of the Center for Global Development, sponsored by the Bill & Melinda Gates Foundation. This report is based on research and analysis conducted under the auspices of RAND Health, a division of the RAND Corporation, in the division's Center for Domestic and International Security. Partial support for this project was provided by gifts from Carol and David Richards and Charles Martin.

Contents

Tables

Summary

Developing countries are facing enormous health problems, notably from infectious diseases such as HIV/AIDS, malaria, and tuberculosis, and lack of access to basic health care, clean water, adequate sanitation, and food. Recognizing the magnitude of these problems, governments, international organizations, for-profit corporations, and nonprofit organizations throughout the world regularly provide both cash and in-kind resources to developing countries to help them address their health needs. In addition, the Millennium Development Goals (MDGs), which call for a dramatic reduction in poverty and marked improvements in the health of the poor by the year 2015, have prompted increased political and financial support. Even so, much more remains to be done if the health needs of developing countries are to be adequately addressed and the MDGs are to be reached (United Nations, 2003, United Nations Development Programme, 2003).

While it is clear that serious resource gaps remain, the exact magnitude and structure of these gaps are ill documented. Furthermore, as health resources flow from ever more actors—including the governments of both developed and developing countries, international organizations, and the private sector—policymakers must have precise, real-time data on these flows in order to identify resource gaps, target assistance, avoid duplication of efforts, and track progress toward the MDGs.

Current Collections of Health Resource Data

A number of entities—including bilateral assistance agencies, multilateral and research/advocacy organizations, and governments of developing countries—are presently involved in significant efforts to track the flow of health resources to and/or within developing countries. We conducted an in-depth evaluation of these existing health resource data collections to determine how each one's data are structured and to assess the extent to which they address the data needs of the global health community.

The data collections we evaluated represent significant efforts on the part of numerous entities to track the health resource flows to and within developing countries. Some of these data collection efforts have been ongoing for decades and were originated for specific purposes, such as long-term trend analysis, which they have served well. There are, however, significant gaps in the data and in the understanding of global health resource flows.

Currently, the available health resource data constitute a patchwork of information at different levels of aggregation and resolution and of varying quality and timeliness that falls short in meeting the needs of the many diverse objectives and organizations that require such data. Another problem is that many of these data collections focus exclusively either on the health resources provided to developing countries by external sources ("external flows") or on the country-level resources expended on health ("domestic flows"); and the few that capture data on both of these essential elements tend to focus on no more than one disease (e.g., AIDS or malaria). In addition, information about the interface between external and domestic flows is lacking, which raises such critical issues as "additionality"—i.e., the degree to which external funds are truly additional to, rather than a substitute for, previously available domestic funds. And finally, many current data collections rely on labor-intensive collection techniques that require extensive planning and the skills of specially trained teams, which can prove burdensome to those providing the data and may be detrimental to the data's accuracy and timeliness.

Because of these drawbacks, the existing data collections are of limited use in addressing key health policy issues, such as resource mobilization and allocation, for which they were not designed to serve. In sum, the collections are

- Not always sufficiently comprehensive
- Sometimes inaccurate
- Often lacking in timeliness and detail.

The result is that policymakers in developing and developed countries alike have no ongoing access to complete, accurate, up-to-date, detailed data on the resources being devoted to health in developing countries. And without these data, none of the parties trying to address the health problems of developing countries has the empirical knowledge required to answer a variety of questions and to inform policy decisions about health resource mobilization and allocation, strategic planning, priority setting, monitoring and evaluation, advocacy, and general policymaking.

Creating a Global Health Resource Tracking System

To provide an up-to-date, comprehensive picture of the health resources available to developing countries, the existing data collections would have to be improved or a new, less burdensome approach would have to be developed. Any new strategy for collecting current, comprehensive data on global health resource flows would have to (1) be designed for the express purpose of tracking global health resources, (2) include methods for collecting the most up-to-date information available (preferably real-time data, whenever available), and (3) rely on data fed directly from transactional sources so as to reduce (perhaps eliminate) the reporting burden placed on data contributors.

A truly global health resource tracking system would begin by identifying all health resources the moment they enter any one of the "streams" contributing to the worldwide flow of such resources and would then follow these resources through all of their "handlers" and "transformations" to the point at which they were finally "provided." Specifically, such a data system would be able to annually identify and assemble information on all planned activities set forth in the budgets of all (including developing) countries and private entities around the world that were designed to address any of the health needs of any developing country. Then, as these planned activities were set into motion, the funds budgeted to pay for them would be tracked as they were first converted into obligations and then into actual outlays/expenditures. The ideal health resource tracking system would seamlessly follow and integrate all cash and in-kind resource streams in real time without double-counting, and would do so without placing a reporting burden on any of the entities involved.

In short, a truly global health resource tracking system would

- Contain valid, detailed data (who, what, where, how much) on all health resources (cash and in-kind) provided last year (expenditures) and this year (obligations) and to be provided next year (budgeted) to all developing countries by all public and private entities in virtually real time without double-counting any resources.
- Impose on any public or private entity no more than a minimal burden in terms of its provision of the information needed to populate the system.
- Readily harmonize with and connect to the existing data systems of receiving countries and all donor entities.
- Be easily accessible via the Web and flexibly searchable by every data element in a variety of languages.
- Enjoy broad ownership, official buy-in, and use, with long-term support from a diversified funding base.

Using Unobtrusive Measures to Track Health Resources

Many global health resource tracking activities rely on information collected through surveys of government, nongovernmental organization (NGO), bank, foundation, organization, or corporate officials about the institutions for which they are responsible. While definitely of value, surveys have distinct limitations as data collection tools: (1) they typically are unable to filter out the subjective perceptions of respondents, and (2) they are "intrusive" and require the time and cooperation of respondents who will receive little, if any, benefit from their effort.

The use of "unobtrusive measures" is an alternative way to collect data that avoids these problems. The most common type of unobtrusive measure is the running record that a government or other entity creates as it conducts its routine business. And since the most common type of running record is a transactional record that memorializes an exchange of money, this approach is ideally suited for tracking the flow of resources among various entities.

Every entity that provides health resources to the world's developing countries maintains records of the resources it provides each year and the recipients of such resources. In the developed countries, international organizations, and NGOs that provide developing countries with cash for purchasing health resources, these records are budgets and/or procurement and disbursement documents. In the entities that provide in-kind health resources to developing countries (e.g., pharmaceuticals), these records are product distribution and/or shipping documents. Once these resources are received by the developing countries and combined with the resources provided by the developing countries themselves, they can be tracked in-country using the internal disbursement and distribution documents maintained by the national, regional, and/or local governments, as well as by the international organizations and NGOs operating internally in these countries.

These routinely generated business records are the unobtrusive measures upon which a global health resource tracking system could, and indeed should, be based. There are two reasons for using these records: Running records are of unparalleled accuracy and cost nothing to collect, and piggybacking on these running records will ensure that the information in the system is virtually real-time data.

There are, however, limitations to the use of unobtrusive measures. For example, the task of accessing and linking data from different large, complex databases with disparate structures and formats can be quite challenging—especially when different countries and organizations have their own ways of organizing and/or maintaining records. In addition, such data are not always accurate, reliable, or valid: Definitions of terms may change from year to year without being noted, archival records can be subject to errors and changes in record-keeping procedures, and sometimes data are altered for political reasons. However, the data obtained through unobtrusive measures can be checked against information obtained from other sources to verify their accuracy (i.e., triangulation).

There are also other challenges associated with using unobtrusive measures. For example, developing countries that have few resources and little institutional capacity may not maintain centralized, electronic records of health resource flows. However, a significant number of countries with large populations and considerable health expenditures and needs (e.g., Brazil, South Africa, India) do have data systems that are likely to be sufficiently advanced for the use of unobtrusive measures to be feasible. In addition, some entities, such as private corporations and foundations, may be unwilling to share information they regard as proprietary. In contrast, information is usually accessible from public entities (e.g., governments, international organizations, NGOs), many of which are required to publicly report financial data. Several other factors can also make the collection and comparison of data from different countries challenging—for instance, different languages and currencies; diverse accounting practices, data collection procedures, and data gathering systems; and dissimilarly structured health care systems.

In short, while it would not be a trivial matter to create and continuously update a global health resource tracking system that employs unobtrusive measures, it appears feasible to do so on a technical level. The open question is whether it is feasible on a political level.

Conclusions

Policymakers and the entities that are providing health resources to developing countries need better and more-reliable information for their decisionmaking. To supply that information, a comprehensive data collection strategy is needed, one that makes it possible to accurately show the resources being brought to bear by all parties—developing countries, developed countries, international organizations, corporations, and private nonprofit organizations—to combat disease and improve health in developing countries. Such a strategy cannot be created without a fundamental rethinking of how to track health resources on a global basis. Furthermore, given both the complexity of the problem and the general lack of data that are complete, accurate, up to date, and detailed, any workable solution is likely to require a great deal of cooperation and commitment on the part of the providers of health resources and the recipients of those resources alike.

Acknowledgments

We wish to thank all of the people who were enthusiastic and cooperative participants in the interviews and Technical Consultation for providing invaluable information about health resource tracking in developing countries: Sono Aibe, Senior Program Manager, The David and Lucile Packard Foundation; Julia Benn, Administrator, Statistics and Monitoring Division, Development Co-operation Directorate (DCD), Organisation for Economic Co-operation and Development/Development Assistance Committee (OECD/DAC); Peter Berman, Professor of Population & International Health Economics and Director of International Health Systems Program, Harvard School of Public Health; Stan Bernstein, Sexual and Reproductive Health Policy Adviser, Millennium Project; Stefano M. Bertozzi, Director, Health Economics, Instituto Nacional de Salud Publica; Karen Cavanaugh, Health Systems Management Analyst, United States Agency for International Development (USAID); Don Creighton, Manager, Global Policy/Corporate Policy & Strategic Management, Pfizer, Inc., Corporate Affairs; Susna De, Coordinator, National Health Accounts Initiative, Partners for Health Reform*plus* (PHR*plus*)/Abt Associates; Paul De Lay, Director, Monitoring and Evaluation, The Joint United Nations Programme on HIV/AIDS (UNAIDS); Tania Dmytraczenko, Health Economist and Associate, PHR*plus*/Abt Associates; Jacqueline Eckhardt-Gerritsen, Project Leader, Resource Flows Project, Netherlands Interdisciplinary Demographic Institute (NIDI); Sally Ethelston, Vice President for Communications, Population Action International; Sarah Ewart, Policy Analyst, Malaria Vaccine Initiative; Katherine Floyd, Stop TB Department, World Health Organization (WHO); Tamara Fox, Program Officer, Population Programs, William and Flora Hewlett Foundation; Joel Friedman, Senior Fellow, Center on Budget & Policy Priorities; Charo Garg, Health Economist, Health System Financing, Expenditure & Resource Allocation, WHO; Amparo Gordillo-Tobar, Consultant on Health Economics and Financing, Pan American Health Organization (PAHO); Pablo Gottret, Senior Health Financing Economist, World Bank; Brian Hammond, Head, Statistics and Monitoring Division, DCD, OECD/DAC; Alison Hickey, Manager, AIDS Budget Unit, Budget Information Service, Institute for Democracy in South Africa (Idasa); John Howe III, President & CEO, Project HOPE; Jose-Antonio Izazola-Licea, Executive Coordinator, Regional AIDS Initiative for Latin America & Caribbean (SIDALAC); Jennifer Kates, Director, HIV Policy, Kaiser Family Foundation; Kei Kawabata, Coordinator of Resource Flows, Expenditures, and Risk Protection Team, WHO; Patience Kuruneri, Senior Adviser, Roll Back Malaria Partnership Secretariat, WHO; Bill Leinweber, Vice President, Research America; Maureen Lewis, Senior Fellow, Center for

Global Development; Eric Lief, independent consultant; Patrick Lydon, Health Economist, Immunization, Vaccines, and Biologicals Department, WHO; Bill McGreevey, Director, Development Economics, The Futures Group International; Emiko Naka, Global Fund to Fight AIDS, Tuberculosis, and Malaria; Paul Nunn, Coordinator, TB/HIV and Drug Resistance, Stop TB Department, WHO; Mead Over, Senior Economist, Development Research Group, World Bank; Ann Pawlicsko, NIDI monitor, United Nations Populations Fund (UNFPA); Rudolphe Petras, Administrator, Statistics and Monitoring Division, OECD/DAC; Ravi P. Rannan-Eliya, Associate Fellow, Health Policy Programme, Institute of Policy Studies; Lisa Regis, UNAIDS; Blair Sachs, Program Officer, Global Health Policy & Finance, Bill & Melinda Gates Foundation; Russ Scarato, Health Economist, USAID; Nina Schwalbe, Director, Public Health Programs, Open Society Institute; Barbara Seligman, Senior Policy Advisor, Bureau of Global Health, USAID; David Sevier, Principal, MAPA Ventures; James Sherry, Vice President, Policy, Research & Advocacy, Global Health Council; Anil Soni, Friends of the Global Fund; Sergio Spinaci, Executive Secretary, Coordination of Macroeconomic & Health Support Unit, Sustainable Development & Health Environments, WHO; Ruben Suarez-Berenguela, Economic Advisor, EquiLAC, National Health Accounts, PAHO; Todd Summers, President, Progressive Health Partners; Ron Waldman, Head of Maternal and Child Health Task Force, and Clinical Professor of Epidemiology, Millennium Project; Veronica Walford, Director, Institute for Health Sector Development (UK); Joseph C. Whitehill, Senior Analyst, International Development, Congressional Budget Office, U.S. Congress; Virginia Yee, Director, Accessible Information on Development Activities (AiDA) Development Gateway, World Bank.

We would also like to thank Catherine Michaud, Senior Research Associate at the Harvard Center for Population and Development Studies, for her involvement in the interviews and Technical Consultation, her advice throughout the preparation of this report, and her insightful and timely review of this report.

We would also like to thank Ruth Levine, Senior Fellow and Director of Programs, Center for Global Development, for sharing her insights on global health resources.

We would also like to thank our RAND colleagues who contributed to this report: Connie S. Moreno, who conducted background research and contributed to the glossary; David M. Adamson, who contributed his considerable writing expertise to the report; Michael Stoto, who was the RAND peer reviewer for the report; Ross Anthony, who provided valuable insights on international health; and Robin Cole, who organized the Technical Consultation.

Abbreviations

AiDA	Accessible Information on Development Activities
AIDS	Acquired Immunodeficiency Syndrome
BIS	Budget Information Service
CARIS	Current Agricultural Research Information System
CDC	Centers for Disease Control and Prevention
CFDA	Catalog of Federal Domestic Assistance
CGD	Center for Global Development
CRIS	Country Response Information System
CRS	Creditor Reporting System
DAC	Development Assistance Committee (of OECD)
DAI	Development Activity Information
DCAS	Development Cooperation Analysis System
DCD	Development Co-operation Directorate
DCPP	Disease Control Priorities in Developing Countries Project
DELSA	Directorate for Employment, Labour and Social Affairs (of OECD)
DFID	(UK) Department of Foreign International Development
DOD	Department of Defense
DOL	Department of Labor
DOTS	Directly Observed Treatment, Short-Course
DPT	Diphtheria, Pertussis, and Tetanus
EC	European Commission
EIU	Economist Intelligence Unit
ENRAP	Electronic Networking for Rural Asia/Pacific Projects
EUROSTAT	Statistical Office of the European Communities
FAADS	Federal Assistance Awards Data System
FCAA	Funders Concerned About AIDS
FPDS	Federal Procurement Data System
FSP	Financial Sustainability Plan
FTF	Financing Task Force (within GAVI)
FY	Fiscal Year
GAVI	Global Alliance for Vaccines and Immunization
GDP	Gross Domestic Product
GFATM	Global Fund to Fight AIDS, Tuberculosis, and Malaria
GKAIMS	Global Knowledge Activity Information Management System
GNI	Gross National Income

GNP	Gross National Product
GRID	Global Response Information Database (Country Response Information System)
HA	Health Accounts
HBCs	High-Burden Countries
HIV	Human Immunodeficiency Virus
HRSA	Health Resources and Services Administration
ICHA	International Classification for Health Accounts
ICPD	International Conference on Population and Development
Idasa	Institute for Democracy in South Africa
IDB	Inter-American Development Bank
IDML	International Development Mark-up Language
IDRC	International Development Research Centre
IEC	Information, Education, and Communication
IMF	International Monetary Fund
IND	Indicator Database (of CRIS)
INDEV	India Development Information Network
INDIX	International Network for Development Information Exchange
INTAL	Institute for the Integration of Latin America and the Caribbean
IRDES	Institut de Recherche et d'Etude en Economie de la Santé
ISIC	International Standard Industrial Classification
ITU	International Telecommunications Union
LAC	Latin American and Caribbean
MDGs	Millennium Development Goals
MoH	Ministry of Health
MTEF	Medium Term Expenditure Framework
NARSIS	Natural Resources Information System
NCU	National Currency Unit
NGO	Nongovernmental Organization
NHA	National Health Accounts
NHExp	National Health Care Expenditure (database)
NIDI	Netherlands Interdisciplinary Demographic Institute
NIH	National Institutes of Health
NORAD	Norwegian Agency for Development Cooperation
NPISH	Nonprofit Institutions Serving Households
NSF	National Science Foundation
NTP	National Tuberculosis Control Program
OA	Official Aid
ODA	Official Development Assistance
OECD	Organisation for Economic Co-operation and Development
PAHO	Pan American Health Organization
PEPFAR	President's Emergency Plan for AIDS Relief
PHN	Population, Health and Nutrition (USAID)
PHR*plus*	Partners for Health Reform*plus*
PPP	Purchasing Power Parity
PQMD	Partnership for Quality Medical Donations

PRISME	Program and Project Information System on Education
PRN	Policy Research Network (Global Health)
PRT	Project Resource Tracking (CRIS database)
RaDiUS	Research and Development in the United States (database)
R&D	Research and Development
RID	Research Inventory Database (CRIS)
SHA	System of Health Accounts
SIDA	Swedish International Development Cooperation Agency
SIDALAC	Regional AIDS Initiative for Latin America & Caribbean
SNA	System of National Accounts
STD	Sexually Transmitted Disease
SWAp	Sector-Wide Approach (SWAp) (programs)
TB	Tuberculosis
UN	United Nations
UNAIDS	Joint United Nations Programme on HIV/AIDS
UNCDF	United Nations Capital Development Fund
UNCTAD	United Nations Conference on Trade and Development
UNDP	United Nations Development Programme
UNESCO	United Nations Educational, Scientific and Cultural Organization
UNFPA	United Nations Population Fund
UNGASS	United Nations General Assembly Special Session
UNICEF	United Nations Children's Fund
UNPOP	United Nations Population Division
USAID	United States Agency for International Development
USDA	Department of Agriculture
WDI	World Development Indicators
WHO	World Health Organization
WHO CHOICE	World Health Organization CHOosing Interventions that are Cost-Effective

Glossary of Terms

Additionality: The concept that new funding for health resources is additional to, and not a substitute for, funds already available for health. The net, rather than the gross, impact after allowances have been made for what would have existed in the absence of the intervention.

Administrative records/data: Information collected, processed, and stored in automated information systems (e.g., enrollment, eligibility, and claims information).

Bilateral donation/funding: Financial resources provided directly by a donor country to an aid recipient country without being passed through a third party organization.

Budget: Quantitative plan of activities and programs expressed in terms of assets, liabilities, revenues, and expenses. An estimate of revenue and expenditures for a specific period.

Commitment (see Obligation): In a financial context, a liability—i.e., a promise or a firm decision to spend money.

Country in transition: A nation whose economy is changing from that of a "developing country" to that of a "developed country."

Data: Factual information.

Database: A collection of factual information organized such that a computer program can quickly select desired pieces of it. An "electronic filing cabinet" that provides a common core of information that is accessible via a computer program. A collection of factual information stored on a computer storage medium, such as a disk, that can be used for more than one purpose.

Data mining: Looking for hidden patterns in a collection of factual information. Looking for previously unknown relationships among the bits and pieces of factual information.

Data tracking system (see Tracking system): An automated network that electronically collects, stores, retrieves, and tracks factual information.

Data weaving: Harvesting factual information from disparate sources with incompatible formats and then connecting the disparate pieces using common embedded codes to produce a complete picture.

Developed country: A nation that has achieved (currently or historically) a high degree of industrialization and that enjoys the higher standard of living made possible by wealth and technology. There is a strong correlation between this status and having democratic institutions.

Developing country: A low- or middle-income nation having per capita gross national product (GNP) and/or income thresholds below a specific level. A nation that has not achieved a significant degree of industrialization relative to the size of its population and that has a low standard of living. There is a strong correlation between this status and high population growth. The term is used for countries that are in the process of developing, but is often also used, euphemistically, for countries that are not.

Direct feed: Digitized, factual information coming straight from the source without interference of any kind. Note that "direct feed" is not the electronic extraction of information from a data system(s) and/or the importation of that information to another data system using a targeted Web crawling mechanism to pull data out of systems.

Disbursement (see Expenditure/outlay): An outlay of cash. The payment of money by cash or check to discharge an obligation or a commitment. The release of funds to a given entity or the purchase of goods or services—the amount thus spent. The actual transfer of financial resources or of goods or services valued at the donor's cost .

Donor: Person or entity that gives or bestows a benefit on another; a giver.

Expenditure/outlay (see Disbursement): The issuance of a check, disbursement of cash, or electronic transfer of funds to liquidate an expense.

Grant: A transfer made in cash, goods, or services for which no repayment is required. A transfer payment from a government to a recipient to help fund a project or activity that does not involve substantial governmental participation.

Health resource(s) (domestic and external): Cash (or its equivalent), products and equipment (including in-kind donations), or services used to address the health care needs of institutions, organizations, and/or individuals.

In-kind resource: A payment in goods or services, as opposed to money.

Interview (see Survey): To have a personal meeting with someone to obtain specific information.

Loan: A transfer of funds for which repayment is required with or without the payment of interest.

Monetary resource(s): Money, cash; cash resources.

Mulilateral donation/funding: Flows of resources from a number of entities that are channeled via an international organization active in helping countries develop their economies and raise their standards of living.

National Health Accounts/National Accounts: The framework for which countries' estimates of spending for health care are constructed. The framework can be considered a two-dimensional matrix having health care providers or products that constitute the health care industry along one dimension, and sources of funds used to purchase this health care along the other dimension. Also, accounts used to trace all the resources that flow through the health system over time and across countries.

Nongovernmental organization (NGO): A private, not-for-profit organization that operates exclusively in one country (national NGO) or in more than one country (international NGO).

Obligation (see Commitment): Budgeted funds that are committed to be spent. An expected expenditure backed by an agreement.

Original data (see Primary data): Factual information that is not derivative or dependent.

Out-of-pocket health expenditure/cost: A direct outlay, including a gratuity or a payment in-kind, of an individual and/or a household to a health practitioner or supplier of pharmaceuticals, therapeutic appliances, or other goods and services whose primary intent is to contribute to the restoration or the enhancement of the health status of the individual or population groups.

Primary data (see Original data): Factual information that is independent, rather than subordinate to or derived from other factual information. First-hand factual information.

Primary mission: The main task with which a person or entity is charged.

Processed data: Factual information that has gone through a series of instructions executed by a computer.

Questionnaire (see Survey): A list of questions used to seek information from a selected group, usually for statistical analysis.

Raw data: Factual information that has not been subjected to a process giving it significance.

Real-time data: Current factual information. A computer term for a data processing system that provides decisionmaking information on a current basis—i.e., at the time a decision needs to be made or while a system user waits for a response.

Recipient: An entity receiving funds—e.g., a developing country's government, a national NGO, or a donor's field office in a developing country.

Reporting burden: The responsibility of periodically furnishing others with financial information to aid in control or decisionmaking.

Resource flows: The creation, transformation, exchange, transfer, or extinction of transactions that affect the amount of economic value of a unit or sector. Resource flows involve changes in the volume, composition, or value of the transactions that affect the amount of economic value of a unit or sector.

Resource tracking: Observing, collecting, and following transactions that can add to the amount of economic value of a unit or sector.

Retrospective data: Factual information that looks back over the past.

Running records: Related data items that are gathered on a continual basis.

Secondary data source: A source of factual information that is not the primary source of factual information. A subordinate source of factual information.

Secondary mission: A task or purpose that is not the primary task or purpose. A subordinate task or purpose.

Survey: A systematic collection and analysis of data relating to the attitudes, living conditions, opinions, etc., of a population, using a representative sample of that population.

Tracking system (see Data tracking system): An information network that reveals how and/or from where the items of factual information contained within the system were obtained.

Transactional records/data: Factual information about the day-to-day events in a business that change its financial position and/or earnings.

Unobtrusive measure: A record routinely created by a government or other entity as it goes about/conducting its regular business. Information collected without special intrusion. Unconsciously provided information.

References for Definitions

Barron's Accounting Handbook, 2nd Edition, Joel G. Siegel, and Jae K. Shim, Barron's Educational Series, Inc., 1990.

Barron's Dictionary of Computer and Internet Terms, 5th Edition, Douglas Downing, Michael Covington, and Melody Mauldin Covington, Barron's Educational Series, Inc., 1996.

Barron's Finance & Investment Handbook, 3rd Edition, John Downes and Jordan Elliot Goodman, Barron's Educational Series, Inc., 1990.

Bureau of Labor Statistics online glossary, www.bls.gov/bls/glossery.htm.

Cambridge Dictionaries on-line, http://dictionary.cambridge.org/.

Centers for Medicare & Medicaid Services (CMS) online glossary, www.cms.hhs.gov/glossary.

Congressional Budget Office online glossary, www.cbo.gov/showdoc.cfm?index=4032&sequence=14.

"Fact Index," http://www.fact-index.com/.

"The Free Dictionary," http://encyclopedia.thefreedictionary.com/.

Fossum, Donna, et al., *Discovery and Innovation: Federal Research and Development Activities in the Fifty States, District of Columbia, and Puerto Rico*, Santa Monica, CA: The RAND Corporation, 2000.

OECD/DAC Glossary, http://www.oecd.org/glossary.

Oxford English Dictionary, http://dictionary.oed.com/entrance.dtl.

UK Treasury, "The Green Book," http://greenbook.treasury.gov.uk/annex01.htm.

United Nations, Department of Economic and Social Affairs, Statistics Division, http://unstats.un.org/unsd/sna1993/introduction.asp.

United Nations Population Fund, "Financial Resource Flows for Population Activities in 2001." "Webopedia Computer Dictionary," www.webopedia.com

"Wikipedia, the Free Encyclopedia," http://en.wikipedia.org/wiki/Main_Page.

World Health Organization, World Bank, and United States Agency for International Development, *Guide to Producing National Health Accounts: With Special Application to Low-Income and Middle-Income Countries*, Geneva, Switzerland: WHO, 2003.

CHAPTER ONE

The Data Challenge

A growing body of work has documented the dimensions of a global health crisis. AIDS, tuberculosis, and malaria kill more than six million people each year, and the numbers are rising.[1] Millions more die every year from preventable illnesses caused by lack of access to immunizations, poor access to clean water, inadequate sanitation, and malnutrition. The gaps in mortality between rich and poor populations are widening, most notably in Africa, where 35 percent of children are at higher risk of dying today than they were a decade ago and adult mortality has risen since the 1990s because of HIV/AIDS (World Health Organization, 2003). In addition, a global increase in noncommunicable diseases is adding to the daunting challenges already facing many developing countries (World Health Organization, 2003). In recognition of the enormity of these health problems, governments, international organizations, corporations, and nonprofit organizations throughout the world regularly donate both cash and in-kind resources to developing countries to help them address their health needs.

The Millennium Development Goals (MDGs) call for a dramatic reduction in poverty and marked improvements in the health of the poor by the year 2015.[2] Governments in developed and developing countries, aid agencies, and nongovernmental organizations (NGOs) are reorienting their work to address the MDGs (United Nations Development Programme, 2003). A number of multiyear global initiatives are also working to meet the MDGs, including the Global Polio Eradication Initiative; Global Fund to Fight AIDS, Tuberculosis, and Malaria (GFATM); World Health Organization "3 by 5" Initiative; Roll Back Malaria Partnership; Stop TB Partnership; and Global Alliance for Vaccines and Immunization (GAVI). The amount of aid to developing countries is indeed increasing, and major reforms are under way, but much more needs to be done to reach the MDGs (United Nations, 2003; United Nations Development Programme, 2003).

While it is clear that serious resource gaps remain, the exact magnitude and structure of these gaps are ill documented. Furthermore, as health resources flow from ever more parties, including developed and developing country governments, international organizations,

---

[1] Global Fund to Fight AIDS, Tuberculosis, and Malaria, http://www.theglobalfund.org/en/.

[2] The MDGs are the embodiment of the Millennium Declaration, which was unanimously adopted by the member states of the United Nations (UN) at the Millennium Summit in September 2000. The eight MDGs bind countries to join forces in the fight against poverty, hunger, illiteracy, lack of education, gender inequity, child and maternal mortality, disease, and environmental degradation. The eighth goal calls on developed countries to create a "global partnership for development" through increased aid, debt relief, and fair access to their markets and technology. For more on the MDGs, see http://www.un.org/millenniumgoals/.

and the private sector, the need to provide policymakers with precise, real-time data on these flows so that they can identify resource gaps, target assistance, avoid duplication of efforts, and track progress toward the MDGs becomes increasingly critical.

Currently, a number of entities, including bilateral assistance agencies, multilateral and research/advocacy organizations, and governments of developing countries, are involved in significant efforts to track the flow of health resources to and/or within developing countries. (For details, see Chapter Two, Appendix B, and Appendix C.) Some of these data collection efforts have been ongoing for decades and were originated for other purposes, such as long-term trend analysis, which they have served well. However, for purposes such as resource mobilization and allocation (as outlined below), these existing data collections are of limited use because they are

- Not always sufficiently comprehensive
- Sometimes inaccurate
- Often lacking in timeliness and detail.

In addition, many of these data collections focus exclusively either on the health resources externally provided to developing countries ("external flows") or on country-level expenditures on health ("domestic flows"), but not both; and the few that do capture data on both of these essential elements tend to focus on resources devoted solely to one disease (e.g., AIDS). Furthermore, information about the interface between external and domestic flows is lacking, which raises critical issues, such as that of "additionality"—i.e., the degree to which external funds are truly additional to, and not a substitute for, previously available domestic funds. And finally, many current data collections use laborious collection techniques that require extensive planning and specially trained data collection teams, all of which place a large burden on those providing the data.

The result is that policymakers in developing and developed countries alike do not have ongoing access to complete, accurate, up-to-date, detailed data on the resources being devoted to health in developing countries. There thus is a need to create a new, comprehensive strategy for collecting data that accurately shows the resources being brought to bear by all parties—be they developing countries, developed countries, international organizations, corporations, or private nonprofit organizations—to combat disease and improve health in developing countries. And such a strategy cannot be created without a fundamental rethinking of how health resources can be tracked on a global basis.

The Need for Data on Health Resource Flows

Reliable data on the health resources available to developing countries are essential for a variety of purposes, including strategic planning, priority setting, monitoring and evaluation, advocacy, and general policymaking. Without such data, parties trying to address the health problems of developing countries do not have the empirical information they need to make informed decisions about two key health policy issues confronting them: the nature and magnitude of the health resources to be mobilized, and the allocation of health resources. To ensure adequate and predictable flows of health resources to developing countries (mobilization) and to determine the best distribution of health resources within developing countries (allocation), high-quality data on the specific resources flowing into and within the health sector of these countries are needed (Partners for Health Reform*plus*, 2003a).

Over the years, the collection and monitoring of the data on health resources flowing into and within developing countries have come to be known as *health resource tracking*. As noted, health resource tracking is important for answering essential questions, as well as for informing policy decisions about health resource mobilization and allocation. Specific uses of these data include the following:

- *Resource mobilization.* Health resource tracking provides policymakers with the information needed to assess the adequacy of the resources available for health programming and to strategize about ways to increase the availability of these resources. Specifically, the data obtained by tracking health resources are valuable for
  — Assessing the gaps between available and estimated health resource requirements.
  — Providing external donors with information about how and whether the health resources they contribute are additional to (as opposed to substituting for) the health resources available from domestic sources.
- *Resource allocation.* Health resource tracking helps policymakers determine whether scarce health resources are being used effectively within a developing country and whether the distribution of health resources within a country matches that country's priority health programs (e.g., HIV/AIDS, immunization) and population groups (e.g., women, children, indigenous populations). It can also facilitate the implementation of initiatives, such as the Poverty Reduction Strategy plans of various developing countries to reduce poverty, by providing the data with which to monitor their progress, and it can document the resources devoted to achieving the MDGs and other global initiatives (World Health Organization, 2003).

The data generated by health resource tracking systems are critical to optimizing the effectiveness of any new (i.e., additional) health resources that are provided to developing countries and to minimizing any duplication of effort. Organizational decisionmakers are also interested in targeting new resources more precisely to specific geographic regions, population groups (e.g., school-age children, women of child-bearing age), or domains of activity (e.g., condom use). These decisionmakers use health resource tracking data to facilitate both global and in-country coordination of health resource distribution.

Health policy questions and decisions at the country level differ from those at the global level, so the health resource data needed in the two contexts also differ. Specifically, health decisionmakers at the country level need data on the size and type of both the domestic and the external resource flow, as well as on trends; and decisionmakers at global-level organizations need data on the specific contributions being made by all donors, including details about the receiving country, targeted disease, type of intervention, and entity actually receiving the resources. Even though the data needs of the two groups differ, however, they are still closely related. It is therefore important to examine how the parallel processes of global and national health resource tracking are intertwined.

What Are Health Resources?

Defining Health Resources

In this report, we define the term *health resources* as cash (or its equivalent), products and equipment (including in-kind donations), or services used to address the health care needs of institutions, organizations, and/or individuals.[3] While this definition is widely embraced by professionals in the health resource tracking field, it is critical to note that it is *not* used consistently in all major health resource data collections. That is, the definition of *health resources* and what the term encompasses differ from organization to organization and from data collection to data collection. For example, the Organisation for Economic Co-operation and Development (OECD) uses at least three different definitions of *health resources* in the course of conducting its numerous activities.

Specifically, OECD's Development Assistance Committee (DAC) tracks external flows of health resources to developing countries as "aid to health,"[4] whereas OECD's Directorate for Employment, Labour and Social Affairs (DELSA) tracks domestic resource flows within OECD countries as "total expenditure on health."[5] As a consequence, OECD/DAC specifically includes medical education, training, and research in its definition of *aid to health*, whereas OECD/DELSA excludes medical education, training, and research from its definition of *total expenditure on health*.

When the focus turns to national health accounts, however, OECD uses yet another set of measures to determine what constitutes health resources. Specifically, the OECD manual entitled *A System of Health Accounts* (SHA) presents the International Classification for Health Accounts, in which *health resources* is defined, as is the case with OECD/DELSA, as "total expenditure on health."[6] However, what is and is not considered to be under the umbrella of total expenditure on health differs in several important aspects between OECD SHA and OECD/DELSA.

The OECD SHA manual also defines *health resources* in terms of both "public expenditure on health care" and "private expenditure on health care," be it domestic or external

---

[3] In this report, the term *health care needs*—whether in relation to an institution, organization, or individual—is broadly defined to include preventive, curative, palliative, and rehabilitative care.

[4] OECD/DAC defines *aid to health* as including (1) "basic health," which includes basic health care, basic health infrastructure, basic nutrition, infectious disease control, health education, and health personnel development; and (2) "health, general," which includes health sector policy, planning, and programs; medical education, training, and research; and medical (nonbasic) health services (OECD/DAC, http://www.oecd.org/document/44/0,2340,en_2649_34447_24670956_119656_1_1_1,00.html).

[5] OECD/DELSA defines *total expenditure on health* as the sum of expenditures on activities that, through application of medical, paramedical, and nursing knowledge and technology, have the goals of (1) promoting health and preventing disease; (2) curing illness and reducing premature mortality; (3) caring for persons affected by chronic illness who require nursing care; (4) caring for persons with health-related impairments, disability, and handicaps who require nursing care; (5) assisting patients to die with dignity; (6) providing and administering public health; and (7) providing and administering health programs, health insurance, and other funding arrangements (Organisation for Economic Co-operation and Development, 2004).

[6] The OECD SHA manual (Organisation for Economic Co-operation and Development, 2000) defines *total expenditure on health* to include (1) services of curative care, (2) services of rehabilitative care, (3) ancillary services to health care, (4) medical goods dispensed to outpatients, (5) services of prevention and public health, and (6) health administration and health insurance. It specifically excludes from this definition (1) education and training of health personnel; (2) research and development in health; (3) food, hygiene, and drinking water control; (4) environmental health; (5) administration and provision of social services in kind to assist living with disease and impairment; and (6) administration and provision of health-related cash benefits.

to a country. Specifically, the OECD SHA manual defines these public and private expenditure terms as follows (Organisation for Economic Co-operation and Development, 2000):

- *Public expenditure on health care:* Health expenditure incurred by public funds. Public funds are state, regional, and local government bodies and social security schemes. Public capital formation on health includes publicly financed investment in health facilities plus capital transfers to the private sector for hospital construction and equipment.
- *Private expenditure on health care:* Privately funded part of total health expenditure. Private sources of funds include out-of-pocket payments (both over the counter and cost sharing), private insurance programs, charities, and occupational health care.

In short, although there is general consensus about what health resources are, there is no agreement at the operational level about what the term actually encompasses. As a result, it is very difficult to compare the information contained in various collections of health resource data.

Tracking Health Resources—Budget Versus Obligation and Expenditure Information

Some health resource data collections track amounts planned to be spent (i.e., budgets); others track amounts to be drawn down over time (i.e., obligations) or amounts actually expended in a calendar year (i.e., disbursements, expenditures, or outlays). These differ from each other in terms of the information provided and the time at which the information occurs—that is, what is first a budgeted amount becomes an obligated amount of funding that in turn becomes an actual amount of funding expended.

Budgets are a natural point from which to begin tracking health resources, since budgets show where all institutionally provided resources originally came from. Budget execution databases and accounting reports can be used to track decisions made about health resources from the point of formulation to the point of commitment and sometimes disbursement to the awardee (e.g., grantee, contractor). Indeed, well-formulated budgets that take into account the long-term objectives and needs of specific health programs, as well as government spending policies on health care, can be extremely helpful in guiding institutional decisions about out-year health resource allocations. In contrast, statistics that document prior-year spending plans on health resources are of limited use to institutional decisionmakers, as they all too often describe actions that were superseded by events or changed by the effects of subsequent decisions. Consequently, real-time budget data are needed to support the coordination of longer-term health resource allocation decisions as well as near-term health resource mobilization decisions.

While information on the funds actually obligated or expended for health care may be of limited use in allocating and mobilizing these resources, it may provide a more accurate assessment of a health care system's financial status than budget information does, and it may also be useful for long-term trend analysis. That is, even though funds may be budgeted for certain purposes, they may not be committed or spent accordingly. Also, budget information can only be collected from the institutional providers of health resources, such as governments, international organizations, and corporations—not from individual households. In addition, obligation and expenditure data should reflect the actual cost of major disease burdens or epidemics, whereas budget information provides estimates of future needs. Nevertheless, all health resource budget processes will benefit greatly from knowing how much has been obligated and/or expended to deliver individual health care services (Partners for Health Reform*plus*, 2003a).

In short, when tracking health resources, it is important to have information on budgets, obligations, and expenditures because each provides different and important information. Indeed, to obtain an accurate picture of the allocation and mobilization of health resources over time, it is critical to have budget, obligation, and expenditure information from as many as possible of the entities funding health care.

Purpose of This Report

This report has been prepared to provide the background analyses required to identify the relevant parameters for the design and construction of a global health resource tracking system. Specifically, this report examines (1) the purposes and contents of existing health resource tracking systems focused on developing countries, (2) the strengths and limitations of these systems, and (3) the characteristics of a global health resource tracking system that would meet the needs of potential users and address the limitations of current systems.

We conducted a series of extensive interviews with the key people involved in operating and/or managing all current major health resource data collections to understand how these collections are structured and populated, and to assess the extent to which they meet the needs of the global community. During these interviews, we gathered information on the types and the characteristics of health resource data needed to support research, advocacy, and policymaking.

The information from these interviews was combined with the results of extensive research on current health resource data collections to produce a Working Paper entitled "Inventory of Health Resource Data Collections." We used this paper as background material to help frame the discussion at a technical consultation on health resource tracking, as described next.[7]

Technical Consultation on Health Resource Tracking

The RAND Corporation and the Center for Global Development (CGD) convened a technical consultation on health resource tracking on May 10–11, 2004, at the RAND conference facility in Arlington, VA. This consultation was held under the auspices of the Global Health Policy Research Network (PRN), a CGD program sponsored by the Bill & Melinda Gates Foundation. The RAND Corporation is one of the institutional members of the PRN.

Many of the key players involved in providing, receiving, and/or tracking health resources in developing countries attended the technical consultation (see Appendix A for a complete list of attendees). The goal of the consultation was to obtain from specific subject-matter experts in the production and use of resource data both technical guidance and input

---

[7] Information from this RAND Working Paper is in Chapter Two and Appendices B and C.

on how to design a new data framework for tracking cash and in-kind resource flows to the health sector in the developing world.

The objectives of the technical consultation were to

(a) Obtain an up-to-date understanding of the types and the characteristics of data needed to track all of the resources going to global health.
(b) Identify the important gaps in the existing efforts to track health resources that it is hoped would be filled with a new, more comprehensive tracking system.

The consultation was structured to foster an open exchange of information and views among individuals with extensive knowledge of resource tracking issues. It featured a series of interactive sessions consisting of short, formal, introductory presentations followed by ample time for free and open discussion and interaction among the participants. The presentations and discussions focused on the following:

- Policy uses of health resource tracking data
- The definition of the term *health resource*
- The data needs and desires of health resource data users
- The characteristics of a truly global health resource tracking data system
- The strengths and limitations of current health resource data collections
- Future approaches for tracking global health resources.

The substance of the discussions and the preparatory documents provided to the participants form the core of this report, which, along with the results of the consultation, will be used by the Global Health Resource Tracking Working Group convened by PRN to guide the mission, membership, and work plan of the group that is to develop the technical specifications for a future health resource tracking data system. The Resource Tracking Working Group will be tasked with assessing the feasibility of a global health resource tracking data system, devising a blueprint for a global health resource tracking data system, and providing recommendations to the global health community on approaches that might be taken to create a sustainable, effective global health resource tracking data system.

Organization of This Report

Chapter Two presents an overview of all current major health resource data collections and briefly assesses their strengths and limitations. Chapter Three describes the characteristics of a more comprehensive global health resource tracking system, discusses the potential users of such a system, and provides details about an approach for collecting data on health resource flows using unobtrusive measures as an alternative to surveys. Chapter Four concludes our report with a discussion of the implications for further work based on the data needs of the global health community and the currently available data tracking global health resources.

The Glossary, which appears in the front matter, lists and defines the key terms and concepts used in the report. Appendix A lists those who participated in the technical consultation. Appendix B is a spreadsheet containing details of each data collection overviewed in Chapter Two. Appendix C is a detailed inventory of the health resource data collections listed in Appendix B, as well as a brief discussion of several others of some potential relevance. Appendix D lists the people with whom extensive interviews were conducted to obtain information about all current major health resource data collections. Appendix E lists the questions that were asked during the interviews conducted with the key people involved in the operations and/or management of the major health resource data collections.

CHAPTER TWO

Current Collections of Health Resource Data

As noted in Chapter One, many entities around the world are assisting developing countries with their enormous health care needs. Some of these entities, as part of their assistance effort, are also collecting or assembling information that touches on some aspect of the health needs of and health resources available to developing countries. Concomitantly, several of them are helping developing countries set up and maintain a system of national health accounts in order to produce a more accurate picture of the country's specific health needs and the resources required to address them. Because each of these efforts focuses on a specific country, disease, or type of resource, however, the currently available data collections on the health resources available to developing countries are haphazard and fragmented and therefore incapable of being harmonized to create a complete and accurate global picture of the health needs of developing countries. Indeed, since the primary purpose of many of these data collections is to support long-term trend analysis and to ensure that governments and organizations fulfill their promises of assistance (i.e., to provide accountability), much of the available information on global health resources is so dated and/or lacking in detail that it is of little or no use for identifying the current health needs of developing countries and/or targeting the available health resources to where they will do the most good (i.e., to where they will provide critical additionality).

An Inventory of Health Resource Data Collections

This chapter is primarily an inventory of all the presently available, major health resource data collections that track health resource flows to and within developing countries and countries in transition. Specifically, we present a detailed look at the components of each of the major data collections now available. We provide the basic information needed to compare the types of health resource data available in each of the collections, information that can also serve as the basis for identifying overall gaps in the available health resource data. The information provided in this chapter, as well as that in Appendices B and C, served as background material for the technical consultation on health resource tracking that the RAND Corporation and the Center for Global Development (CGD) convened on May 10–11, 2004, in Arlington, VA.

As discussed in Chapter One, we use the term *health resources* to mean cash (or its equivalent), products and equipment (including in-kind donations), or services used to address the health care needs of institutions, organizations, and/or individuals. Consequently, health resources can be funds, products, or services. And as noted specifically in Chapter

One, this definition of *health resources* is widely embraced by professionals in this field but is *not* used consistently in the major health resource data collections described in this chapter. In particular, although all of the data collections in this inventory contain information on the funds devoted to "liquid" health resources (i.e., cash or its equivalent), few of them contain information on in-kind health resources (i.e., health resources provided as services and/or products). It is important to note, therefore, that within the context of this chapter, it was necessary to work with the definitions of health resources actually used by the tracking systems being summarized.

Several organizations have developed and maintain health resource data collections. Indeed, some organizations, such as the Organisation for Economic Co-operation and Development (OECD), Pan American Health Organization (PAHO), and World Health Organization (WHO), have developed and maintain multiple such data collections. The data collections detailed in this inventory come in two different formats: assembled in databases and assembled in reports. All but one of them, a database, gather some primary data. Thus, both types of data presentations described here—databases and reports—represent significant data collection efforts by the sponsoring organizations.

The health resource databases and reports featured in this inventory could be organized in several ways—for example, by primary versus secondary data collections, type of funding reported, countries or regions covered, or substantive area of health tracked. After much consideration and the discovery that data on the flow of health resources to and within developing countries are of central value to policymakers and donors, we decided that the best way to subdivide the health resource data collections was according to whether they feature data on (1) donor aid (external flows), (2) country-level expenditures (domestic flows), or (3) both. Collections that feature data on country-level expenditures were further subdivided into those that specifically use the National Health Accounts (NHA) methodology and those that use other methods of data collection. The health resource data collections presented in this chapter are thus grouped as follows:

- *Data on donor aid.* Collections that specifically track donor aid going to developing countries.
- *Data on country-level expenditures/activities.* Collections that specifically track country-level expenditures and/or activities.
  - *Data on country-level expenditures/activities: National Health Accounts, National HIV/AIDS Accounts, and other disease-specific subanalyses.* Collections that specifically track country-level expenditures and/or activities using the NHA methodology.
  - *Data on country-level expenditures/activities: Other.* Collections that specifically track country-level expenditures and/or activities using other methods of data collection.
- *Data on donor aid and country-level expenditures/activities.* Collections that track both donor aid going to developing countries and country-level expenditures and/or activities.

Table 2.1 lists the health resource data collections in terms of type, name, and sponsoring organization. All collections listed are described briefly in this chapter; more-detailed

Table 2.1
Health Resource Data Collections

Type of Collection	Name	Supporting Organization
Data on donor aid	CRS (Creditor Reporting System)—Database on Aid Activities	Organisation for Economic Co-operation and Development (OECD)/Development Assistance Committee (DAC)
	AiDA (Accessible Information on Development Activities)	Development Gateway Foundation
	Report on HIV/AIDS Grantmaking by U.S. Philanthropy	Funders Concerned About AIDS (FCAA)
	U.S. Government Funding for HIV/AIDS in Resource Poor Settings	Kaiser Family Foundation HIV Policy Program
	Global Funding for HIV/AIDS in Resource Poor Settings	
Data on donor aid and country-level expenditures/activities	Resource Flows Database	United Nations Population Fund (UNFPA)/Joint United Nations Programme on HIV/AIDS (UNAIDS)/Netherlands Interdisciplinary Demographic Institute (NIDI)
	Global Tuberculosis Control: Surveillance, Planning, Financing	World Health Organization (WHO)
Data on country-level expenditures/activities: National Health Accounts, National HIV/AIDS Accounts, and other disease-specific subanalyses	OECD Health Data	OECD/Directorate for Employment, Labour and Social Affairs (DELSA) Health Policy Unit
	National Health Accounts	WHO
	Health Accounts/National Health Accounts	Pan American Health Organization (PAHO)
	National Health Accounts; National Health Accounts Subanalyses	Partners for Health Reform*plus* (PHR*plus*)/Abt Associates
	National HIV/AIDS Accounts	SIDALAC (Regional Initiative on HIV/AIDS for Latin America and the Caribbean)
Data on country-level expenditures/activities: Other	World Development Indicators	World Bank
	National Health Care Expenditure (NHExp) Database; Data Base of Trade in Health Related Goods and Services in the Americas	PAHO
	Idasa Budget Information Service (BIS) Budget Briefs and Reports	Institute for Democracy in South Africa (Idasa)
	Immunization Financing Database	Global Alliance for Vaccines and Immunization (GAVI)
	Country Response Information System (CRIS)	UNAIDS

information on them is provided in Appendix B (as a spreadsheet) and in Appendix C. The collective strengths and limitations of these data collections are discussed at the end of this chapter.

Methodology

We conducted an in-depth evaluation of existing health resource data collections to determine how the data are structured in each one and to assess the extent to which they address the sizable data needs of the global health community. The collections in this inventory were selected because they are currently the major sources of information available for tracking health resources in developing countries. Some of the data collections detailed here are in the form of databases; others are assembled as reports. Some of the databases serve as the basis for annual reports on health resource flows in developing countries.

Information for this inventory was obtained using a variety of methods. Specifically, we conducted a series of extensive interviews with the key people involved in the operations and/or management of the major health resource data collections (see Appendix D for the list of interviewees). All interviewees were asked about the health resource data collections at their organizations: What data are collected, from whom, and how? Who uses the data collected and for what purposes? Are there identifiable gaps in the data being collected and/or reported on health resources? Are there additional health resource data collections that should be included in the inventory? Appendix E lists the specific questions asked during these interviews.

The information obtained in the interviews, which often involved numerous iterations to verify specific details, was supplemented with information gained directly from detailed analyses of the databases and reports themselves. Further supplementation was in the form of information gleaned from critical examinations of relevant reports, user's manuals, and Websites. As a last quality assurance step, a final draft report of the descriptions of the data collections was sent to each of the individuals responsible for the data collections to allow them to comment on or correct any of the information contained in the report.

Data on Donor Aid

Creditor Reporting System (CRS)—Database on Aid Activities

Description

The Creditor Reporting System (CRS) is the online database developed and maintained by the Development Assistance Committee (DAC), which is the unit of OECD with primary responsibility for carrying out OECD's work involving cooperation with developing countries. The specific purpose of CRS is to collect timely information and comprehensive statistics on the official and private aid going to developing countries, and to make these statistics available to OECD/DAC members so that they can provide better aid to these countries. CRS is "the keeper" of the official statistics of the official development assistance (ODA) and official aid (OA) provided by OECD/DAC members to developing countries.[1] CRS

---

[1] The DAC List of Aid Recipients, used to help measure and classify aid and other resource flows originating in DAC countries, is divided into two parts: Part I consists of "traditional" developing countries, and Part II consists of "more advanced" eastern European and developing countries. "Official development assistance" (ODA) is aid, in the form of grants or loans, given to countries and territories on Part I of the DAC List of Aid Recipients. Aid to the countries on Part II of the list is recorded separately as "official aid" (OA). (The DAC List of Aid Recipients is available online at http://www.oecd.org/document/45/0,2340,en_2649_34469_2093101_1_1_1_1,00.html.)

contains both textual and numerical information on individual aid transactions (e.g., specific projects). The primary users of the database are the DAC members themselves.

DAC also maintains a companion database to the CRS, the DAC Database on Annual Aggregates, which provides aggregate data on the volume, origin, and types of aid and other resource flows to over 180 recipients (developing countries and countries in transition). In short, the DAC Database provides aggregate information on aid flows, and the CRS provides detailed information at the project level.

Data

CRS data are gathered via questionnaires completed and submitted quarterly by all OECD/DAC members. Non-OECD/DAC members can submit comparable information to CRS on a voluntary basis. CRS supplements these data with information on the loan transactions of World Bank, Inter-American Development Bank (IDB), African Development Bank, and International Fund for Agricultural Development.

The dollars reported in CRS are commitments (obligations)—i.e., the face value of the activity on the date a grant or loan agreement is signed with the recipient. Cancellations and/or reductions of earlier years' commitments are not reported in CRS.[2] In recent years, data at the activity level on actual disbursements (outlays) have also been made available online, but these are not as complete as the data on commitments because they are obtained for only 70 to 80 percent of donors.

CRS does not contain data on some or all of the aid provided to developing countries by the Commission of the European Communities, multilateral organizations (i.e., the United Nations Development Programme [UNDP]),[3] and nongovernmental organizations (NGOs). It also does not include data on bilateral aid flows from non-OECD/DAC members (e.g., China); aid flows from the core budgets of NGOs; foreign direct investment, unguaranteed bank lending, and portfolio investment; contributions made by OECD/DAC members to multilateral agencies;[4] and loans made out of funds held in the recipient country. In-country resource flows are difficult to follow, and information on them is mostly obtained through case studies.

Accessible Information on Development Activities (AiDA)

Description

Accessible Information on Development Activities, or AiDA, as it is more commonly known, is an online database. Hosted and maintained by the Development Gateway Foundation, it is the largest single source of integrated information on development activities. AiDA selectively catalogues information on development activities that is made available on the Websites and from the internal information systems of donors, implementing agencies, and content aggregators that participate in the AiDA project. AiDA's purpose is to address the

---

[2] From the User's Guide to the online aid activity database (CRS), http://www.oecd.org/document/50/0,2340, en_2649_34469_14987506_1_1_1_1,00.html.

[3] Many multilaterals have their own internal classification systems and do not use the same codes as DAC to classify their activities. The UN, for example, has its own codes, which do not necessarily match DAC's.

[4] Contributions by DAC members to multilateral agencies are not available in CRS but are available in aggregate form in the DAC Database on Annual Aggregates.

demand, particularly among AiDA members, for timely and reliable information about who is doing what development activities where and what kind of results they are getting.

Development Gateway Foundation is a nonprofit organization whose mission is to increase knowledge sharing, improve public sector transparency and government efficiency, enhance the effectiveness of development assistance, and build local capacity. The AiDA project builds on the work of the International Network for Development Information Exchange (INDIX) and the International Development Mark-up Language (IDML) initiative.[5] The latter provides users with a common Web interface that allows them to integrate information from multiple Web-based sources into a single, consolidated report.

Data

Organizations that participate in AiDA share information from their Websites and/or internal information systems about their planned, current, and completed development assistance activities, as well as any development assistance programs that they fund, execute, and/or help to implement. AiDA users can search for and retrieve this information using a variety of criteria, such as country, sector or topic, funding organization, or status of activity. The scope of information in AiDA varies by source, as does the frequency of updates, which come monthly, quarterly, or annually, depending on the schedules of the participating organizations.

The primary sources of donor information in AiDA are the Inter-American Development Bank, the International Development Research Centre (IDRC) Development Research Information System, International Monetary Fund, John D. and Catherine T. MacArthur Foundation, Natural Resources Information System, United Kingdom Department of Foreign International Development, United Nations Capital Development Fund, United Nations Population Fund, United States Agency for International Development, and World Bank. CRS, with information from 23 members and major multilateral organizations, shares aggregated donor information through AiDA, while aggregated information by region, country, or theme is shared via AiDA by the Fundacion Acceso, Current Agricultural Research Information System, Electronic Networking for Rural Asia/Pacific Projects, El Salvador Country Gateway, Global Knowledge Activity Information Management System, India Development Information Network, International Telecommunications Union, Program and Project Information System on Education, and Web-based Information System for Agriculture and Sustainable Rural Development.[6]

Although AiDA is currently the largest single source of information on development activities, its information is neither comprehensive nor up to date. For example, AiDA contains almost 500,000 records of development activities, but these records may describe a strategic objective, a program, a project or subproject, technical assistance, or a study grant. And because the information in AiDA is not consistently detailed, it is impossible to distinguish among these different levels/types of activities. The coverage and quality of the information are improving, however, as more organizations participate in AiDA.

---

[5] AiDA, http://aida.developmentgateway.org/AidaAbout.doc.

[6] http://aida.developmentgateway.org/AidaSourcesDesc.do.

Report on HIV/AIDS Grantmaking by U.S. Philanthropy

Description

The *Report on HIV/AIDS Grantmaking by U.S. Philanthropy*, which is the most recent report available from Funders Concerned About AIDS (FCAA), provides information about the HIV-related contributions from all sectors of U.S. philanthropy, including foundations, public charities, and corporations (Funders Concerned About AIDS, 2003).[7] It is a practical tool for helping grantmakers develop and sustain their own efforts, as well as for helping others to understand philanthropists' critical role in the response to the HIV/AIDS epidemic. The objective of this report is to improve the understanding and working relationships between the two groups in order to improve the flow of resources to HIV/AIDS programs.

FCAA does not itself make grants or provide any form of direct assistance. It is an association of grantmakers whose purpose is to mobilize leadership and resources to address this pandemic. FCAA has made available a series of publications that research and analyze the data on HIV-related grantmaking from all sectors of U.S. philanthropy.

Report

FCAA gathers, organizes, and reports data on U.S. grant commitments (as opposed to actual spending) to HIV/AIDS programs by calendar year. Multiyear grants are counted fully in the year in which the funds are initially committed, rather than in the years in which the funds are spent. This practice is consistent with that used for the data collections of the Foundation Center; the Funders Network on Population, Reproductive Health and Rights; and several other groups that are primarily made up of grantmakers (Funders Concerned About AIDS, 2003).

FCAA distributed a survey to 78 grantmakers in July 2003, requesting specific information about their HIV/AIDS-related funding allocations in 2001 and 2002. When data were not directly available from the grantmaking entity, FCAA collected information from other sources. FCAA also compared the data it obtained from the surveys and its other research with Foundation Center statistics for 2001 and 2002. The final 2003 dataset for FCAA covers a total of 407 grantmakers for 2001 and 2002, although the 2002 data are less comprehensive and final than the 2001 data.

The FCAA report for 2003 includes information on the HIV-related contributions of foundations, public charities, and corporations. The report also describes in-kind donations from the corporate sector and that sector's sponsorship of related workplace programs, such as awareness and prevention. In addition, the report lists the top 50 HIV/AIDS grantmakers and describes the regional and international distributions of private, U.S.-based grants.

FCAA does not track the activities of faith-based organizations, governments, and international institutions involved in HIV-related grantmaking. However, it is working in partnership with other organizations to support a broad coalition effort aimed at mapping the full multisectoral response to HIV/AIDS (Funders Concerned About AIDS, 2003). These other organizations include the Joint United Nations Program on HIV/AIDS (UNAIDS), World Bank, Kaiser Family Foundation, Global Business Coalition on HIV/AIDS, and European HIV/AIDS Funders Network.

---

[7] The report is available online at http://www.fcaaids.org/about/.

U.S. and Global Funding for HIV/AIDS in Resource Poor Settings

Description

The Kaiser Family Foundation HIV/AIDS Policy Program collects primary data on U.S. funding and gathers secondary data on global funding for HIV/AIDS in developing countries. Its purpose is to provide data on the HIV/AIDS epidemic (including policy reports, fact sheets, and survey data) and information on media partnerships, journalist training programs, and public education campaigns. In addition, the program includes online news summaries and information resources provided through a free online resource. The Kaiser Family Foundation describes itself as a source of independent information for policymakers, the media, the health care community, and individuals and families concerned with major health care issues.[8]

Among the most recent of its publications are two policy briefs. The first, "U.S. Government Funding for Global HIV/AIDS Through FY 2005," provides detailed data on U.S. government funding for the global HIV/AIDS epidemic through FY 2004 and on the budget request for FY 2005 (Kates and Summers, 2004). The second, "Global Funding for HIV/AIDS in Resource Poor Settings," summarizes data on the resources being applied to fight the HIV/AIDS epidemic in developing countries, including support from bilateral and multilateral donor governments, private-sector entities (e.g., support from corporations, foundations, and NGOs), and the developing countries' own governments (Summers and Kates, 2003a).

Report

Because the methods the Foundation's HIV/AIDS Policy Program uses to collect data on U.S. government funding and other funding (e.g., that of other major bilateral donors, affected country governments, and foundations) are different, we discuss them separately here.

U.S. Government Funding. The Kaiser Family Foundation has collected data on U.S. government funding specifically earmarked for HIV/AIDS programs in resource-poor settings from FY 1986, when the U.S. government first began funding global HIV/AIDS activities, through the President's budget proposal for FY 2005. The most recent policy information from the Foundation presents an overview of these data broken down by whether the funding was for bilateral programs; for contributions to the Global Fund to Fight AIDS, Tuberculosis, and Malaria (GFATM); or for international research.

Most of the data on U.S. government funding of HIV/AIDS represents funds specifically designated (earmarked) for global HIV/AIDS programs or initiatives in either bill text or final report language of appropriations legislation (Kates and Summers, 2004). Data are available at the program level for the federal departments/agencies responsible for the most U.S. international HIV/AIDS activities, including the Centers for Disease Control and Prevention (CDC), United States Agency for International Development (USAID), Department of State, National Institutes of Health (NIH), Department of Defense, Department of Labor, and Department of Agriculture. Additional information is obtained from CDC and NIH regarding their own funding of international HIV/AIDS research and their estimates of future funding, as well as from a variety of other primary sources, including congressional appropriations legislation, federal budget documents, reports and estimates from

---

[8] Henry J. Kaiser Family Foundation, http://www.kff.org/about/index.cfm.

government agencies, and analyses by the U.S. Congressional Research Service (Summers and Kates, 2003a).

The Kaiser Family Foundation's data cover most U.S. international activities and contributions to multilateral organizations, as well as the President's Emergency Plan for AIDS Relief (PEPFAR). Information on some kinds of support is not available, such as agency funds not earmarked by Congress and U.S. general support to the UN (which has its own organizations addressing the epidemic). Also, because many programs have become increasingly integrated, disaggregated data on funding are not consistently collected.

Other Global Funding. The Foundation also gathers data on the estimated and/or actual funding from donor governments, governments of affected countries, multilateral organizations, and private-sector donors (i.e., foundations, corporations, and NGOs). Currently, these data contain the estimates of current and future funding needs from 1996 through 2007.

UNAIDS is the primary source of data on funding from non-U.S. governments. Included are estimates of HIV/AIDS-related spending by developing countries' own national governments. Estimates of related grantmaking by foundations and corporations come from FCAA; estimates of actual disbursements by foundations and large international NGOs come from UNAIDS.

Data challenges identified by the Foundation include the lack of a uniform reporting system, delays in reporting, aggregation of data into broader categories (e.g., reproductive health and sexually transmitted diseases), the inability to distinguish budgeted funding levels from actual disbursed amounts, and actual inconsistencies between reported budgeted funding levels and actual disbursements.

Data on Donor Aid and Country-Level Expenditures/Activities

Resource Flows Database

Description

The United Nations Population Fund (UNFPA) has collected data and reported on flows of international financial assistance to population activities since 1980 and on domestic resource expenditures in developing countries since 1994. The most recent report containing this information is *Financial Resource Flows for Population Activities in 2002* (United Nations Population Fund, 2004).[9] Since 1997, the Netherlands Interdisciplinary Demographic Institute (NIDI) has been under contract to UNFPA to collect data for the resource flows reports. Working with UNFPA, NIDI created a Resource Flows Database of both donor and domestic expenditures on population activities. In 1999, UNAIDS joined the UNFPA/NIDI collaboration.

The purpose of the Resource Flows Project is to establish a refined annual data collection, monitoring, and information dissemination system on global financial flows for population activities in developing countries and countries in transition. The Resource Flows Database includes expenditure data on population activities, including family planning services; basic reproductive health services; basic research, data, and population and devel-

---

[9] Reports are available online at http://www.resourceflows.org/index.php/articles/c77/.

opment policy analysis; and STD and HIV/AIDS—including prevention, care and treatment, and support/social mitigation data.[10]

Data

The Resource Flows Project collects and reports data on international population assistance and domestic expenditures for population activities in developing countries and countries in transition. Data are collected through mail surveys and questionnaires, case studies, and the OECD/DAC database. There are annual donor surveys of approximately 180 donors, biennial domestic questionnaires, and approximately 15 case studies that measure the financial resource flows within developing countries and describe the system of health sector financing and policy. To avoid double-counting, the data are collected at the project level but reported at an aggregate level.

The Resource Flows Project does not collect data on such private-sector expenditures as private insurance and out-of-pocket spending. The database is not available online. All data gathered for it are treated as confidential and remain the property of UNFPA; data for HIV/AIDS expenditures are jointly the property of UNFPA and UNAIDS. The data collecting challenges for this project include sorting out data from integrated programs and timeliness. These challenges stem from the fact that although data are collected for the previous fiscal year, the figures are not released and the report is not published for two years because of the delay in collecting the expenditures and clearing the data from all respondents.

Global Tuberculosis Control: Surveillance, Planning, Financing

Description

In March 2004, WHO released its eighth annual report on global tuberculosis control: *Global Tuberculosis Control: Surveillance, Planning, Financing* (World Health Organization, 2004a).[11] The purpose of this series of annual reports is to chart progress in global tuberculosis control and in implementing DOTS (Directly Observed Treatment, Short-Course), the internationally recommended tuberculosis control strategy. The current report contains data on the notification of tuberculosis cases and treatment outcomes from all national tuberculosis control programs that have reported to WHO. It also contains an analysis of plans, budgets, expenditures, and constraints on DOTS expansion for the 22 high-burden countries (HBCs) for tuberculosis.[12]

In 1991, the World Health Assembly ratified the targets for global tuberculosis control by year 2000. These targets, which included successful treatment of 85 percent of detected smear-positive tuberculosis cases and detection of 70 percent of all smear-positive cases, were not met by 2000, so the target year has been reset to 2005. The purpose of these

---

[10] The definition of *population activities* used by UNFPA/UNAIDS/NIDI covers the "costed population package" classification system as outlined in paragraph 13.14 of the Programme of Action of the International Conference on Population and Development (ICPD) held in Cairo in 1994 and the key targets set out in the UNGASS Declaration of Commitment on HIV/AIDS (http://www.resourceflows.org/index.php/articles/49).

[11] Report available online at http://www.who.int/tb/publications/global_report/en/.

[12] The HBCs for tuberculosis are Afghanistan, Bangladesh, Brazil, Cambodia, China, Democratic Republic of Congo, Ethiopia, India, Indonesia, Kenya, Mozambique, Myanmar, Nigeria, Pakistan, Philippines, Russian Federation, South Africa, Thailand, Uganda, United Republic of Tanzania, Vietnam, and Zimbabwe.

data is to assess progress toward the 2005 targets. The current report contains eight consecutive years of data.

Report

As of 2002, the annual report on global tuberculosis control has included financial analyses. Data were collected directly from countries via a one-page questionnaire included in the annual WHO data collection form. For the most recent report, the National Tuberculosis Control Program (NTP) managers were asked to complete two tables—one about the NTP budget for FY 2003 and the related funding and funding gaps, and another about NTP expenditures and the funding source for them for FY 2002. Data from GFATM proposals, WHO CHOICE (CHOosing Interventions that are Cost-Effective) estimates of the costs of bed days and outpatient visits, and published and unpublished costing studies were also used.

A total of 201 countries reported to WHO on their strategies for tuberculosis control and on tuberculosis case notifications and/or treatment outcomes (World Health Organization, 2004a). Financial data were received from 123 countries, 77 of which provided complete data on 2003 budgets (including 17 HBCs), and 74 of which provided complete, disaggregated expenditures for 2002 (including 15 HBCs) (World Health Organization, 2004a).

Since the financial analysis for tuberculosis control began in 2002, WHO has continued to identify new areas to track. For example, WHO would like to track annual budget and expenditures for multi-drug-resistant tuberculosis and HIV-associated tuberculosis, and has added questions to the survey for the 2005 report to address this.

Information is only obtained on "total grants," so information on individual grants is not available, which makes it impossible to look at trends in grants from particular donors and to determine the major donors. NTP managers will be asked to complete a separate column on the tables for the 2005 report for funds from GFATM, since it is a major donor to the HBCs.

Contributions given to the health sector as sectorwide grants or loans are not reported because it is difficult to determine the portion that is specifically used for tuberculosis. Since such disease-specific financing makes it difficult to determine where these types of funds originate, they are usually reflected as government contributions.

Data on Country-Level Expenditures/Activities: National Health Accounts, National HIV/AIDS Accounts, and Other Disease-Specific Subanalyses

General Description

National Health Accounts (NHA) are an internationally accepted methodology for determining a nation's total health expenditure patterns, including public, private, and donor spending (Partners for Health Reform*plus*, 2003a).[13] NHA address four basic sets of questions (World Health Organization, 2002): Where do resources come from? Where do resources go? What kinds of services and goods do resources purchase? Who benefits from re-

---

[13] The NHA approach is not yet standardized, so methodologies and definitions differ by country. A guide developed by WHO, World Bank, and United States Agency for International Development (2003) represents an effort to harmonize and standardize the different approaches for producing NHA.

sources? NHA attempt to answer these questions by showing the flow of financing from a source of funding to a particular use, to a user of that expenditure, or to beneficiaries following a standard classification of health expenditure (World Health Organization, 2002). Basically, NHA show where the money comes from and where the money goes.

NHA were implemented in a number of middle- and low-income countries in the mid- to late 1990s. To date, approximately 70 countries around the world have conducted NHA, and more than 50 NHA have been conducted in low- and middle-income countries (Partners for Health Reform*plus*, 2003b). However, many countries have conducted no more than one study. Currently, of the countries conducting NHA, only one-third do so on a regular, sustained basis (Partners for Health Reform*plus*, 2002).

NHA describe the flow of resources specifically within the health sector. They track total expenditures on health, which encompass all expenditures for activities whose primary purpose is to restore, improve, and maintain health for the nation and for individuals (Partners for Health Reform*plus*, 2003b). Health expenditures are commonly defined as all expenditures for prevention, promotion, rehabilitation, and care; population activities; nutrition; and emergency programs for the specific objective of improving or maintaining health. Health includes both the health of individuals and the health of populations (Hjortsberg, 2001). Total expenditures on health are a combination of both public outlays and private outlays on health (World Health Organization, 2004b).

NHA are essentially a standard set of tables that organize and present health expenditure information in a simple format (Partners for Health Reform*plus*, 2003a). Production of NHA requires extensive data collection from various ministries, donors, households, providers, and industry groups (e.g., private insurers, employers, pharmaceutical companies). Data come from a wide variety of sources, including government records (e.g., budget reports, tax reports, import and export statistics); other public records (e.g., ministry of health annual reports, financing and regulatory agency reports, NGO reports, academic studies, international agency reports); insurer records; provider records; and household surveys (World Health Organization, 2003). Information is obtained from multiple sources to triangulate (i.e., verify) data.

Several organizations are actively involved in the development, collection, dissemination, and analysis of NHA, including OECD, WHO, PAHO, and Partners for Health Reform*plus* (PHR*plus*). These organizations act as facilitators for country efforts and provide technical assistance and sometimes funding. WHO, PAHO, and PHR*plus* have worked collaboratively in many of the almost 70 countries that have conducted NHA. In addition, WHO, PAHO, and OECD assemble, organize, and cross-check country data and make them accessible to the wider public.

The flexibility of the NHA framework also makes it possible to analyze data on targeted populations or disease-specific activities, such as health expenditures related to child health or HIV/AIDS (Partners for Health Reform*plus*, 2003b). HIV/AIDS expenditures have been tracked using National HIV/AIDS Accounts in Latin America and the Caribbean with the support of the Regional AIDS Initiative for Latin America and the Caribbean (SIDALAC).[14] PHR*plus* has helped countries in East, Central, and Southern Africa to con-

---

[14] National HIV/AIDS Accounts are based on NHA methodology but are not necessarily a subanalysis of NHA. In the majority of countries that have conducted them, National HIV/AIDS Accounts are stand-alone exercises. SIDALAC has developed these accounts in the 22 countries in which it has worked.

duct NHA subanalyses to track expenditures on HIV/AIDS, malaria, and reproductive health, and WHO is also currently using NHA methodology to measure disease-specific expenditures.

The work of OECD, WHO, PAHO, and PHR*plus* on NHA is described in more detail below. National HIV/AIDS Accounts and the use of NHA methodology for disease-specific expenditure analyses are also discussed.

OECD Health Data

Description

OECD Health Data 2004 is the name of an electronic database containing key aspects of the health care systems of the Organisation for Economic Co-operation and Development's (OECD's) 30 member countries.[15] The database was developed jointly by the Health Policy Unit of OECD's Directorate for Employment, Labour and Social Affairs (DELSA) and the Institut de Recherche et d'Etude en Economie de la Santé (IRDES), the objective being to provide a tool that would help health researchers and policy advisors in governments, the private sector, and the academic community to carry out comparative analyses and draw lessons from international comparisons of diverse health care systems. The Health Policy Unit focuses on facilitating both cross-national studies of the performance of OECD health systems and member country exchanges about financing, delivery, and management of health services.

Data

The OECD Health Policy Unit has been publishing health statistics since the mid-1980s. OECD Health Data 2004 is the 13th edition of this interactive database, which covers over 1,200 indicators, spanning 1960 to 2002, and contains some estimates for 2003 and selected long time series from 1960 onward. Demographic, economic, and social contexts are noted, and the data are broken down by category, as follows: health status, health care resource, health care utilization, expenditure on health, health care financing, social protection, pharmaceutical market, nonmedical determinants of health, demographic references, and economic references. Each category is broken down into further levels of detail.

Information about expenditures on health and health care financing in the database generally follows the framework set out in the OECD manual *A System of Health Accounts* (Organisation for Economic Co-operation and Development, 2000). This manual provides an international standard for reporting health expenditures and, among other things, proposes a common boundary for health care. However, OECD member countries are currently at different stages in implementing the system, and not all OECD members use this OECD manual to report health expenditures. Therefore, the data in the OECD Health Data 2004 database have varying levels of comparability (Organisation for Economic Co-operation and Development, 2004). Some countries closely follow the OECD system, some use "locally produced health accounts" that may or may not be comparable, and some rely on national accounts for estimating health expenditure. In one instance, the data are OECD Secretariat

---

[15] The OECD member countries are Australia, Austria, Belgium, Canada, Czech Republic, Denmark, Finland, France, Germany, Greece, Hungary, Iceland, Ireland, Italy, Japan, Korea, Luxembourg, Mexico, Netherlands, New Zealand, Norway, Poland, Portugal, Slovak Republic, Spain, Sweden, Switzerland, Turkey, United Kingdom, and United States.

estimates based on the OECD National Account database. The database does document the definitions, national sources, and estimation methods for each country.

World Health Organization (WHO) National Health Accounts

Description

Since the early 1960s, the World Health Organization (WHO) has collected and analyzed health expenditure data.[16] WHO's goal is to promote the best possible health for all people of the world, and this data collection is an effort to assist in meeting that goal. Over the past five years, WHO has developed a systematic effort to measure resource flows in the health systems. One of the principal products of this effort has been the *World Health Report*, an annual publication providing selected measured ratios and levels of expenditure on health in all WHO member countries.[17] The report includes NHA indicators on total expenditures on health, broken down into public and private expenditures, with additional detail for selected indicators. Data on external resources are also included.

Another product of the effort is WHO's NHA Website. Newly launched in 2004, it offers technical information and support for those conducting NHA, country-specific estimates of health expenditures, and other useful information, such as the ratios available in WHO's *World Health Report* and the absolute values and sources of information for such macro-variables as gross domestic product, general government expenditures, and average official and international dollar exchange rates.[18] Other resources, most notably an NHA database, are being developed.

WHO also builds the capacity of countries to generate health expenditure information through training workshops and direct technical assistance. In addition, WHO, World Bank, USAID, and other partners worked together for three years to produce the *Guide to Producing National Health Accounts: With Special Application to Low-Income and Middle-Income Countries* to provide assistance to countries embarking on the task of measuring their national health expenditures (World Health Organization, World Bank, and United States Agency for International Development, 2003).

Data

WHO's *World Health Report* and its NHA Website provide data on all financing agents and external resources in WHO's 192 member states. The report covers 16 specific indicators, including total expenditure on health as a percentage of gross domestic product, general government expenditure on health as a percentage of total expenditure on health, prepaid and risk-pooling plans as a percentage of private-sector expenditures on health, and how these relate to exchange rates.[19]

---

[16] With the support of WHO, Abel-Smith conducted the first major national studies of health expenditures in developing countries. For more information on these original studies, see Abel-Smith, 1963 and 1967.

[17] Report available at http://www.who.int/whr/en/.

[18] WHO NHA Website is http://www.who.int/nha/en/.

[19] WHO also collects data on more than 50 indicators regularly and on more than 1,000 when they are available, as well as on such dimensions of resource flows as expenditures on pharmaceuticals, hospitals, and inpatient care that have been collated but are not yet available.

Data for NHA estimates come from a wide variety of sources, such as existing reports and national statistical projects, NHA reports, government and other public records, insurer records, provider records, and household surveys (World Health Organization, 2004b). International reports are used to verify data from national reports. WHO also works very closely with OECD, using OECD data where appropriate. The NHA database is a work in progress that will include data collated from several different national and international sources and reports. Data will be consolidated, triangulated, and harmonized in the NHA framework, using international standard classifications and in agreement with national accounts standard procedures.

Approximately 70 countries have conducted NHA to date, and many other countries are beginning them. Many, however, failed to follow up after the initial study, which precludes monitoring and analysis of trends. The ideal system would have a continuous flow of data, instead of a single NHA study for a special interest group, such as donors. The great challenge is to ensure that the collection, compilation, and reporting of health expenditures is done on a routine basis and is sustainable.

Pan American Health Organization (PAHO) Health Accounts/National Health Accounts

Description

Established in 1902, the Pan American Health Organization (PAHO) is an international public health agency whose objective is to improve the health and living standards of the people of the Americas. It is WHO's regional office for the Americas. The Health Accounts (HA) and NHA that PAHO compiles are estimates of total national spending on health, health care services, and national health care systems. PAHO provides technical assistance to countries and maintains regional databases on national health care expenditures and on international trade in health related goods and services. PAHO also provides technical support and guidance to those developing pilot studies based on new and innovative health accounts approaches.

PAHO began including a section on resources in health in its flagship publication, *Health Conditions in the Americas*, in 1994 (Pan American Health Organization, 1994). The most recent report in this series, *Health in the Americas, 2002 Edition*, contains information from 1997 through 2000 (Pan American Health Organization, 2002). In addition, PAHO's Regional Core Health Data Initiative has an online table generator system that allows users to conduct searches on 108 essential health indicators, including health expenditure, for 48 countries and territories of the Region of the Americas from 1997 through 2003.[20]

Data

HA/NHA include public-sector budget data; information on private, out-of-pocket spending, which usually comes from analyses of household survey data; and data on other types of private spending, including expenditures by employers for insurance contributions and direct delivery of health services to workers. Specific sources of data vary from country to country. NHA information in PAHO's *Health in the Americas* series is for all health combined. Country studies on national health care expenditure and financing issues may be based either on

---

[20] PAHO's Regional Core Health Data Initiative Table Generator System is available at http://www.paho.org/English/SHA/coredata/tabulator/newTabulator.htm.

country-specific concepts, definitions, and accounting procedures, which are more relevant to national policy debate, or on existing international standards, which are more relevant to national health systems expenditure and financing patterns.

By June 2003, most Latin American and Caribbean countries had prepared HA/NHA at least once. However, eight countries, mostly in the Caribbean, had yet to do so. In addition, the approaches and methodologies used for HA/NHA estimates vary widely within the region. The institutions involved in making these estimates also vary, although the majority are ministries of health, statistical bureaus, and central banks. Also, more disaggregated data are needed, and additional resources would be needed to prepare them. There are no systematic data on NGOs and nonprofit institutions serving households (NPISH), and information on private health insurance is difficult to obtain.

Partners for Health Reform*plus* (PHR*plus*) National Health Accounts

Description

Partners for Health Reform*plus* (PHR*plus*), a flagship project of the USAID Population, Health and Nutrition Center, has provided support and technical assistance to countries preparing NHA reports for the past eight years. It focuses on building capacity and institutionalizing NHA in developing countries, and it provides a variety of innovative NHA-based analyses.[21] The program's purpose is to strengthen health policy and systems in developing countries and countries in transition. It provides technical assistance to USAID in health care reform, health policy, management, health financing, and system strengthening. In addition, it addresses community participation, infectious disease surveillance, and information systems for managing and delivering appropriate health services, and it conducts health systems research, implements performance monitoring and results tracking, and provides training and capacity development. PHR*plus* is responsible for strategic documentation and transfer of experiences in health policy and systems strengthening.

Report

PHR*plus* works in over 25 countries spanning four regions of the world. It uses information from a variety of sources—studies from ministries of health and finance and from universities, government budgets, surveys and questionnaires (including household surveys), and donor reports—to provide detailed information reports for NHA. These help track the flow of health resources, starting with the funding sources, continuing with those who distribute the funds, and going all the way to the services provided to individuals. This use of multiple sources makes it possible to cross-check the findings.

At times PHR*plus* has to rely on estimates of expenditures because government reports lack sufficient detail, and it sometimes has to look to the local level because some national governments are decentralized. In addition, data on out-of-pocket expenditures by households are often not available, and information from organizations in the private sector is difficult to obtain because they are not required to make their spending information available to the public.

Aside from providing overall views of health systems, PHR*plus* also contributes to NHA subanalyses related to HIV/AIDS, malaria, and reproductive health. Furthermore,

---

[21] PHR*plus*, http://www.phrplus.org/focus_new8.html.

WHO, along with other partners, including PHR*plus*, has initiated a process to standardize disease-specific subanalyses. PHR*plus* is also collaborating with SIDALAC on the tracking of NHA HIV/AIDS expenditures. These two organizations started from different perspectives, but they have arrived at remarkably similar methodologies and are working to map the two together. PHR*plus* is also collaborating on HIV/AIDS subanalyses with a number of other organizations, such as USAID, WHO, and UNAIDS.

Regional AIDS Initiative for Latin America and the Caribbean (SIDALAC) National HIV/AIDS Account

Description

The estimation of national AIDS expenditures—National HIV/AIDS Accounts—in 20 countries in Latin America and the Caribbean is one of the main activities of the Regional AIDS Initiative for Latin America and the Caribbean (SIDALAC).[22] These accounts are the result of "systematic, periodical and exhaustive accounting of the expenditures and financing from the public and private sectors that are directed to the prevention and treatment of people with HIV/AIDS" (Regional AIDS Initiative for Latin America and the Caribbean, 2001). Their main purposes are to influence policy formulation and decisionmaking and to improve the allocation of resources for HIV/AIDS.

SIDALAC was implemented by the Mexican Health Foundation with funding from World Bank. In 1996, UNAIDS came on board as a cosponsor with World Bank. Currently, this initiative is part of UNAIDS and is cosponsored by the United Nations Children's Fund (UNICEF), UNDP, UNFPA, United Nations Educational, Scientific and Cultural Organization (UNESCO), WHO, and World Bank.

Data

SIDALAC tracks both money and services (if there are no records of money spent for services, the cost is estimated) and both health- and non-health-related HIV/AIDS information. It also tracks private, public, and international expenditures. Data are collected through interviews, surveys (although not typically household surveys because of their high cost), and primary sources. SIDALAC depends on the information already available in a country.

SIDALAC is interested in capacity building; it provides hands-on training so that people can set up continuous information systems on resource tracking. SIDALAC is also attempting to standardize the collection and presentation of data. Its presentation is similar to that of OECD SHA and WHO National Health Accounts but has different identification of functions and services for HIV/AIDS

SIDALAC has collected good information on most Latin American countries. It has a sequence of two to four years of resource tracking for most countries and six to seven years for some. The data are not as good for Caribbean countries, where there are more difficulties in capacity building. While most of the information SIDALAC collects is very detailed, different levels of detail are presented in the various reports that SIDALAC prepares. For example, the overall report on all countries is less detailed than the reports on the individual countries. National AIDS program authorities have the most-detailed figures.

---

[22] http://www.sidalac.org.mx/english/home.html.

Data on Country-Level Expenditures/Activities: Other

World Development Indicators (WDI) Database

Description

World Development Indicators (WDI) is World Bank's premier annual statistical report about development. The most recent report, *World Development Indicators 2004*, includes approximately 800 indicators in 87 tables, organized in six sections: World View, People, Environment, Economy, States and Markets, and Global Links. The tables cover 152 economies and 14 country groups, with basic indicators for a further 55 economies. The print edition of *WDI* provides a current overview of data from the past few years. Time-series data from 1960 and onward are available on CD-ROM or online.[23]

Data

WDI Online, available via paid subscription, provides direct access to 575 development indicators, with time series for 208 countries and 18 country groups from 1960 to 2003, where data are available (2003 data are available for selected indicators only). World Bank provides free access to WDI Online through Data Query, which offers a segment of the WDI database.[24] Data Query contains five years of data (1998 to 2002) for 54 indicators for 208 countries and 18 groups.

The primary data collectors for WDI are usually national statistical agencies, central banks, and customs services.[25] Differences in the methods and conventions used by the primary data collectors may have given rise to significant discrepancies over time, both among and within countries (World Bank, 2004). And the quality of the national data may be severely compromised by delays in data reporting and the use of old surveys as the base for current estimates (World Bank, 2004).

Many developing countries lack the resources for training and maintaining the skilled staff and obtaining the equipment needed to measure and report demographic, economic, and environmental trends in an accurate and timely way (World Bank, 2004). World Bank is working with bilateral and other multilateral agencies to fund and participate in technical assistance projects aimed at improving statistical organization and basic data methods, collection, and dissemination (World Bank, 2004). In addition, even though discounts are offered to residents in developing countries, database subscription costs may be prohibitive for some potential users.

National Health Care Expenditure (NHExp) Database

Description

PAHO developed and maintains the National Health Care Expenditure (NHExp) Database, which is a collection of regional data on comparable international indicators of national health care expenditures.[26] Information is presented in two ways: as graphs and tables pro-

---

[23] See http://www.worldbank.org/data/wdi2004/index.htm.

[24] Available at http://devdata.worldbank.org/data-query/.

[25] For the past two years, World Bank has largely used WHO NHA figures in its WDI.

[26] PAHO Website, http://newweb.www.paho.org/English/DPM/SHD/HP/nhexp-datab-intr.htm.

viding snapshots of the data by different categories and groups of countries, and as a database with estimates from 1980 through 1998 for the Americas.

Data

The NHExp Database contains estimates from 48 Latin American and Caribbean countries and territories on public and private expenditures on health. It also contains time series of macroeconomic variables commonly used for deriving national health expenditure indicators and projections, including per capita expenditures, share of health expenditures as a percentage of gross domestic product or gross national income, income-expenditure elasticity, and conversion to purchasing power parity.

Most countries in the region keep data on central-government health expenditures in some form or other. These figures are often produced by national finance authorities and ministries of health for their own internal analysis, as well as for sharing with international agencies. Expenditures at other levels of government (state, provincial, municipal, etc.) are less well documented but are becoming increasingly important in the region. In addition, the data on social security health expenditures vary significantly from country to country in terms of quality and availability and are often years out of date.

Finally, private expenditures on health are relatively undocumented, with no data available for a large percentage of the countries in the region. These expenditures encompass household payments; corporate health expenditures; and the health expenditures of community, religious, and charitable organizations, and other NGOs.

Data Base of Trade in Health Related Goods and Services in the Americas

Description

The Data Base of Trade in Health Related Goods and Services in the Americas, another PAHO activity, provides statistics on international trade in health related commodities in the Americas (Pan American Health Organization and World Health Organization, 2003). It presents estimates of the value of total exports and imports of health related goods and commodities for Canada, United States, and countries of Latin American and Caribbean countries for 1994 through 2000. It also specifically tracks the value of the exports and imports of two broad components of the international trade in health related products: "pharmaceutical, medicinal chemical and botanical products," and "medical and surgical equipment and orthopedic appliances." PAHO's report entitled *Data Base of Trade in Health Related Goods and Services in the Americas* (Pan American Health Organization and World Health Organization, 2003) is available on the PAHO Website.[27]

Data

The main source of data is the Trade Statistics System for the Western Hemisphere, which focuses on import and export statistics. This database, also known as DATAINTAL, consists of programs and databases that allow users to query the data and obtain current and historical trade data in a table format that can be printed or imported into other programs.[28]

---

[27] http://www.paho.org/English/DPM/SHD/HP/trade-datab.htm.

[28] DATAINTAL is available at http://www.iadb.org/intal/ingles/bdi/i-dataintalweb.htm.

DATAINTAL had two developers—the Institute for the Integration of Latin America and the Caribbean (INTAL), in Buenos Aires, Argentina, and the Unit of Statistics and Quantitative Analysis—both of which are units of the Department of Integration and Regional Programs of the Inter-American Development Bank (IDB). The database was designed to meet the needs of decisionmakers, researchers, and analysts concerned with international trade.

INTAL collects trade data from official government organizations that produce national trade statistics and from international organizations. INTAL began collecting trade data in 1984, mainly for internal use by the IDB; and in 1990, it began distributing the data to foreign trade research and promotion organizations in several Latin American countries. The first DATAINTAL version in CD-ROM format was distributed in 1998.

The information in PAHO's database covers only 1994 through 2000. The only year for which information on all 29 countries is included is 1997, so 1997 is used as the reference year for the data.

Institute for Democracy in South Africa (Idasa) Budget Information Service (BIS) Budget Briefs and Reports

Description

The Institute for Democracy in South Africa (Idasa) Budget Information Service (BIS) uses data and budget information from the South African government to analyze revenue and expenditure effects on the lives of low-income, poor, and vulnerable communities. BIS performs issue-based and sector analyses of public spending on HIV/AIDS, health, education, social welfare, human resource and infrastructure development, and local government finance, as well as research on policy and budget allocations affecting vulnerable groups, such as children and women. The objective of this independent research is to enhance the role of civil society organizations in their pro-poor and rights-based advocacy work, to inform parliamentarians in their oversight and monitoring of government departments, to engage government officials, and to influence and advocate budget decisions.[29]

Report

BIS is composed of several units/projects that track public spending on health care in South Africa. One of these, the BIS Children's Budget Unit, has as its main objective research and dissemination of information on the South African government's budgeting for children. It has published several books focused on government spending on children in five key sectors: health, education, welfare, policing, and justice.

Another unit, the BIS Sector Budget Analysis Unit, began in 1995 with a mapping of the new South African intergovernmental system. Its focus at that time was on analyzing government budget allocations and implementation, but it recently broadened its scope to include information that will provide a more comprehensive overview of the impact of public spending on the lives and well-being of poor people and to respond more swiftly to requests for budget information and research in the health, education, and welfare sectors.

The BIS AIDS Budget Unit provides research on and performs analysis of the government's annual HIV/AIDS budget. In November 2003, this unit published a report entitled *Budgeting for HIV/AIDS in South Africa: Report on Intergovernmental Funding Flows for*

---

[29] Idasa, http://www.idasact.org.za/bis/.

an Integrated Response in the Social Sector, which examines provincial capacity and spending procedures for HIV/AIDS programs and gives recommendations on the most-effective ways to channel funds to the provinces to fight the epidemic (Hickey, Ndlovu, and Guthrie, 2003). A companion document to the main report, "Where Is HIV/AIDS in the Budget? Survey of 2002 Provincial Social Sector Budgets," identifies HIV/AIDS specific allocations in provincial education, social development, and health department budgets (Ndlovu, 2003). The AIDS Budget Unit is also coordinating an international comparative analysis of HIV/AIDS expenditure and budgeting in ten countries to compare how governments are funding the fight against HIV/AIDS and to build capacity for HIV/AIDS budget analysis in the participating countries.[30]

Immunization Financing Database

Description

In July 2004, the Immunization Financing Database, a comprehensive database on immunization spending and financing that was developed by the Global Alliance for Vaccines and Immunization (GAVI) Financing Task Force (FTF), became available online with information from 22 countries.[31] The FTF began working on this database in November 2001 with the support of a team of external technical experts. This database focuses on providing information about the baseline for and trends in immunization spending and financial flows.

Data

The Immunization Financing Database provides information about the baseline for and trends in immunization spending and financial flows. Its purpose is to bring about an increased understanding of the inadequate funding for meeting the vaccine and immunization needs of the poorest countries and to identify strategies to improve the capacity of governments, donors, and development banks to finance these needs.

The information in the database is derived from the detailed data on past and future costing and financing that countries submit in their Financial Sustainability Plan (FSP) to GAVI at the midpoint in their funding from the Vaccine Fund.[32] All eligible countries are required to prepare an FSP and provide annual updates. Data are made available in the database after the GAVI's independent review committee has reviewed and accepted the FSP and after the immunization financing database team has reviewed and analyzed the data.[33]

The FSPs include detailed information by cost category and funding source. The cost category includes such recurrent items as vaccines, injection supplies, and training, and such capital items as vehicles and buildings. Retrospective data on costing and financing are required for two years, including a year before GAVI and the Vaccine Fund (baseline year). Prospective data are required for two periods (about eight years). A costing, financing, and gap analysis tool has been developed to assist countries in preparing this information.

---

[30] The ten countries participating are Nicaragua, Argentina, Ecuador, Chile, Mexico, Namibia, Botswana, Mozambique, Kenya, and South Africa.

[31] The Immunization Financing Database is available online at http://www.who.int/immunization_financing/data/en/.

[32] The Vaccine Fund is a financing mechanism designed to help GAVI achieve its objectives by raising new resources and swiftly channeling them to developing countries.

[33] WHO Immunization Financing, http://www.who.int/immunization_financing/data/about/availability/en/.

Countries are asked to report only the source of financing closest to the end use. This means that funds from bilateral donors to multilateral agencies, to sector-wide approach (SWAp) programs, and to national treasuries for budget support are not attributed to the donor countries.[34] In addition, the FSP focuses on program-specific costs, so the data do not account for the national government's contribution to key inputs, such as personnel and facilities, which are shared across multiple health programs.[35]

Country Response Information System (CRIS)

Description

UNAIDS, the main advocate for global action on HIV/AIDS, developed the Country Response Information System (CRIS) to house information collected on indicators, resources, and scientific research relating to HIV/AIDS. The purpose of CRIS is to facilitate the systematic collection, storage, analysis, retrieval, and dissemination of information on a country's response to HIV/AIDS (Joint United Nations Programme on HIV/AIDS, 2003). CRIS provides a structure that countries can use to collect information relative to the epidemic, the response, and the effects. This information includes epidemiological information; strategic planning, costing, and coordination capacities; budget allocations to AIDS programming and other resource flows; and project implementation rates.[36] CRIS, which will be operational in more than 100 countries by 2005, allows direct country-to-country exchanges of information.

Data

CRIS includes a core of standardized information on the HIV/AIDS situation and the response in participating countries. It has three databases: the Indicator Database (IND), the Project Resource Tracking (PRT) database, and the Research Inventory Database (RID). IND, the first component of CRIS to be operational, supports the collection and analysis of local indicators of the HIV/AIDS epidemic. PRT, released in August 2004, allows financial tracking of projects and programs, thus facilitating improved monitoring and evaluation of the national response to HIV/AIDS. RID, currently being field-tested, focuses on enhancing collaboration among decisionmakers and program planners, researchers, research institutions, and funding agencies in order to strengthen the research capacity of developing countries and to enhance the role of research in informing responses to the epidemic.

The country-level CRIS will be complemented by a Global Response Information Database (GRID). Selected data from CRIS for all countries will be housed centrally in GRID by the UNAIDS Secretariat. Data from local CRIS systems will be aggregated and presented on the GRID Website, along with tools to facilitate report creation and to aid those pursuing more-detailed analyses of global data from CRIS. GRID will be constructed so that data updated at the national level in CRIS will be reflected on the global site on a regular basis. GRID will allow data searches across countries and will maximize links with other information systems of the UN system and other strategic partners.

---

[34] WHO Immunization Financing, http://www.who.int/immunization_financing/data/about/limitations/en/.

[35] WHO Immunization Financing, http://www.who.int/immunization_financing/data/about/limitations/en/.

[36] UNAIDS, http://www.unaids.org/EN/in+focus/monitoringevaluation/country+response+information+system.asp.

Examples of Other Types of Databases

Several donors maintain databases that track their own activities. These databases usually contain specific information about the projects/programs that these donors fund. Some of these databases—for example, World Bank's Projects Database and the GFATM Funded Programs Database, both of which are described below—are online, searchable, and publicly available.

There are also several databases that contain specialized information. UNFPA and RH Interchange collect data on contraception; IMS Health, Partnership for Quality Medical Donations (PQMD), UNICEF, WHO, United Nations Conference on Trade and Development (UNCTAD), DATAINTAL, and ECRI (formerly the Emergency Care Research Institute) track pharmaceuticals and medical equipment.

World Bank Projects Database

The Projects Database provides basic information on all World Bank lending projects since 1947, when the bank started operations.[37] It was created to help make the bank's lending more transparent to the public and its partners, and to encourage broader participation in the projects the bank finances. The database can be searched by country, region, sector, priority/goal, or theme. Searching by sectors or by themes provides access to the health related projects funded by World Bank.

Global Fund Funded Programs Database

The Funded Programs Database contains information about grant commitments and disbursements of Global Fund grants.[38] This database can be searched by region, country, funding round, two-year amount, and disease. Information about funding amounts and the text of the full grant proposals are also available.

Quality of Data in Current Health Resource Data Collections

The health resource data collections in this inventory, which are described briefly above and in detail in Appendix C, represent significant efforts on the part of numerous entities to track health resource flows to and within developing countries. These collections provide valuable information about the overall trends in donor aid to, as well as financial flows within, the health sector in developing countries. Some of these data collection efforts have been ongoing for decades and were originated for specific purposes, such as long-term trend analysis, which they have served well.

The health resource data collections described in this inventory have contributed significant information on the health resources available to developing countries. Collectively, however, they have limitations in that they

---

[37] The Project Database is available at http://web.worldbank.org/WBSITE/EXTERNAL/PROJECTS/0,,menuPK:115635~pagePK:64020917~piPK:64021009~theSitePK:40941,00.html.

[38] The Funded Programs Database is available at http://www.theglobalfund.org/en/funds_raised/commitments/.

- Are far from comprehensive;
- Lack critical detail;
- Are not timely; and
- Have accuracy problems.

In addition, most of these collections track either health resources at the donor level or actual expenditures at the country level, but not both. The few that do capture data on both levels tend to focus on the resources going to a specific disease rather than tracking all health resources. Moreover, even when the collections are viewed in combination, there are significant gaps in the data and in the knowledge available on the global flow of health resources to and within developing countries.

We detail the data quality and the strengths and limitations of current health resource data collections next.

Frequency of Data Collection and Period Covered

The existing data collections vary as to how often data are collected. Data for most of the collections are gathered annually, although CRS collects some data quarterly, and AiDA collects some monthly. The frequency with which data are collected for NHA, National HIV/AIDS Accounts, and NHA subanalyses conducted by PAHO, PHR*plus*, and SIDALAC depends on the country in question, since some of the countries conduct NHA studies annually, and others have conducted only one, without doing any follow-ups. The NHA data published by WHO in its *World Health Report* are updated continuously and published annually.

The existing data collections also vary in terms of the period they cover. AiDA contains data as current as 2004, making it the collection with the most up-to-date data publicly available on development activities by international donors. The Kaiser Family Foundation's most recent report contains data on FY 2004 funding, as well as data on the HIV/AIDS funding requested by the President in the U.S. federal budget for FY 2005. Several other data collections—CRS, WDI, Immunization Financing Database, and CRIS—provide data for 2003.

Two of the data collections also provide prospective data. The Idasa BIS Budget Briefs contain Medium Term Expenditure Framework (MTEF) data for 2005 to 2006.[39] The GAVI Immunization Financing Database contains data on future resource requirements and funding gaps, which means data on all the remaining years with Vaccine Fund support and on the years immediately after the Vaccine Fund support ends.

Four of the data collections also contain extensive historical data. The NHA database developed by WHO contains data for certain indicators from 1950 through 2003. Only the data from 1995 through 2001, however, are currently made available to the public. UNFPA's report on population assistance, *Global Population Assistance Report 1982–1988* (United Nations Population Fund, 1989), contains data on international population

---

[39] The MTEF reconciles bottom-up estimates of the costs of carrying out policies, both existing and new, with top-down estimates of aggregate resources available for public expenditure. It is "medium term" because it provides data on a prospective basis, for the budget year (n+1) and for the following two years (n+2 and n+3). MTEF is a rolling process, repeated every year, aimed at reducing the imbalance between what is affordable and what the government ministries demand (http://www.undp.org.vn/projects/vie96028/whatis.pdf).

assistance by major donor category dating back to 1952. Beginning with 1982, data are also available by country. The online and CD-ROM versions of World Bank's WDI database contain data from 1960 through 2003. The CRS database developed by OECD/DAC contains data dating from 1967 through 2003, with data from 1973 onward available online.

Timeliness of Data

The data available on health resources need to be more current. At present, there is a sizable lag between when data are collected and when they are available for use in a database or report. This is particularly true of data collections that report expenditure information, such as NHA, the Resource Flows Database, WDI, NHExp Database, Immunization Financing Database, and UNAIDS CRIS. The information on health resource flows in these data collections typically is at least one year old, and most often it is two years old. In 2004, in recognition of the need for more-current data, UNFPA/UNAIDS/NIDI began collecting information on or making estimates of the year's health resource expenditures, as well as projecting next year's health resource expenditures. AiDA also contains some information on current year spending, the Kaiser Family Foundation report on U.S. government funding of HIV/AIDS includes information on next year's budget proposal, and Idasa Budget Briefs contain projections for both next year and the year beyond.

How Data Are Acquired

The primary way of gathering data on health resources is to administer surveys or questionnaires to government, NGO, bank, foundation, organization, or corporate officials to find out about the institutions for which they are responsible. Those using this method are OECD/DAC for data in CRS; UNFPA/UNAIDS/NIDI for data in the Resource Flows Database; WHO, PAHO, PHR*plus*, and SIDALAC for their NHA, National HIV/AIDS Accounts, and NHA subanalyses; WHO for its report on global tuberculosis control; and FCAA for its report on HIV/AIDS grantmaking. The organizations conducting NHA, National HIV/AIDS Accounts, and NHA subanalyses (i.e., WHO, PAHO, PHR*plus*, and SIDALAC) also extract data from national and international reports on national health expenditures and from household surveys to obtain information on out-of-pocket spending for health care. In addition, SIDALAC compiles data from receipts and ledgers for its National HIV/AIDS Accounts. The Kaiser Family Foundation extracts data from appropriations legislation, legislative report language, U.S. agency estimates, and other official government budget reports to determine U.S. government funding of HIV/AIDS. In a similar manner, it extracts data from UNAIDS, FCAA, and other studies to determine global funding for HIV/AIDS. Idasa extracts the vast majority of the data it uses to prepare its Budget Briefs and other reports from national and provincial budget documents of the South African government. While most data are extracted manually, the Development Gateway Foundation extracts data electronically from the Websites of participating organizations to populate AiDA. UNAIDS is the only entity currently putting in place a system that electronically gathers data directly from partner countries on their HIV/AIDS activities, using both predetermined and free fields, on an ongoing basis.

Primary Versus Secondary Data

Of all the health resource data collections described in this inventory, AiDA is the only one that does not contain some primary data. All of AiDA's data are secondary, pulled from the Websites of its participating organizations. The Kaiser Family Foundation's "Global Funding for HIV/AIDS in Resource Poor Settings" report relies heavily on secondary data provided by UNAIDS, but it also uses a variety of primary data sources for information on the U.S. government. Most of the other data collections contain some, although less, secondary data. The data collections that only contain primary data are CRS, the Immunization Financing Database, CRIS, and the Database of Trade in Health Related Goods and Services in the Americas.

Responding/Reporting Entities

Every health resource data collection gathers data from a number of respondents and/or entities. For example, because CRS and AiDA track donor aid to developing countries, the organizations providing them information include bilateral and multilateral donors and development banks. And the NGOs and private foundations that are partners with AiDA also provide funding information to the database. In contrast, NHA track a nation's total health expenditures, including public, private, and donor spending, so NHA data come from all entities that fund national health care, including national governments (e.g., ministries of health), NGOs, households, providers, and industry groups (e.g., private insurers, employers, pharmaceutical companies).

Both the Resource Flows Database and the *Global Tuberculosis Control* report track donor aid going to developing countries and country-level expenditures and/or activities. The Resource Flows Database collects data from national governments, bilateral and multilateral donors, NGOs, development banks, and private foundations. In contrast, data for the *Global Tuberculosis Control* report come from three main sources: NTPs, GFATM, and the WHO CHOICE Website.

Because the FCAA *Report on HIV/AIDS Grantmaking by U.S. Philanthropy* focuses exclusively on donor aid from the private sector, FCAA collects the information for its report from private and corporate foundations in the United States, as well as from the Foundation Center and similar sources.

In several instances, there are no respondents or reporting entities—the data are gathered from existing documents. For example, Kaiser Family Foundation extracts its information on U.S. funding of HIV/AIDS from U.S. government documents. Similarly, much of the information in the Idasa Budget Briefs is extracted from national and provincial budget documents, while the rest comes from interviews with South African government officials.

Granularity of Data

Another major gap in current health resources information is the lack of detailed data, which are essential if truly informed and effective decisions are to be made about the distribution and use of health resources. At present, many of the major health resource data collections, including the OECD World Health Data and World Bank WDI, contain only aggregate data. And the collections that do contain detailed data do not all use the same level of detail—some contain data on individual projects, some on line items, and still others on functions. Consequently, it is very difficult to make comparisons.

The lack of disaggregated data also makes it difficult to address two important issues: how to measure the additionality of specific health resources, and how to separately track health resources that are part of integrated or sectorwide programs. Neither of these issues can be addressed without a level of detail that is not currently available in most health resource tracking data. Donors are interested in knowing whether, as well as how, their contributions are "additional" to resources coming from domestic sources, and the answers cannot be determined without data on the specific use of both donor and domestic funds. Likewise, the specific recipients and uses of health resources that are part of integrated and sectorwide programs are not generally reported, which makes it difficult to track the flows of these resources.

Type of Funding Reported

Information on health resource funding is reported in one of three ways: (1) as an amount contained/reported in a budget (i.e., "requested" funding), (2) as an obligation or commitment (i.e., "agreed upon" funding), or (3) as a disbursement, an expenditure, or an outlay (i.e., "actual" funding). These types of funding are related in a linear manner in that a budget amount is converted to an agreed-upon amount of funding that eventually becomes the actual amount of funding transferred. Because of this linear transformation, however, the three types of funding are not comparable for any given year.

In light of what we have just said, it is important to note that AiDA reports funding all three ways, depending on the type of funding used in the original data obtained from the participating organization. The Kaiser Family Foundation reports on U.S. and global funding for HIV/AIDS provide data on both budget amounts and obligations. The WHO report on global tuberculosis control and the Idasa Budget Briefs report funding in terms of both budget amounts and expenditures. The CRS reports funding amounts in both commitments and disbursements/expenditures. The FCAA *Report on HIV/AIDS Grantmaking by U.S. Philanthropy* reports funding amounts as commitments. And finally, all of the other health resource data collections report funding amounts as disbursements/expenditures/outlays.

Countries/Regions Covered

A number of health resource data collections contain data on countries located throughout the world: CRS, the Resource Flows Database, AiDA, the Kaiser Family Foundation reports on global funding for HIV/AIDS, WDI, CRIS, WHO NHA, PHR*plus* NHA, and the WHO report on global tuberculosis control.

In contrast, SIDALAC National HIV/AIDS Accounts contain data on health care expenditures for countries in Latin America, the Caribbean, Ghana, and Burkina Faso. PAHO NHA, NHExp Database, and Database of Trade in Health Related Goods and Services in the Americas also contain data for Latin America and the Caribbean, as well as for the United States and Canada.

In addition, PHR*plus* has conducted NHA Subanalysis for HIV/AIDS in Kenya, Rwanda, and Zambia, and has studies under way elsewhere. And while the Idasa Budget Reports focus on budgeting for HIV/AIDS in South Africa only, the Idasa AIDS Budget Unit is coordinating an international comparative analysis of HIV/AIDS expenditures and budgeting in Nicaragua, Argentina, Ecuador, Chile, Mexico, Namibia, Botswana, Mozambique, Kenya, and South Africa. Two of the data collections feature U.S.-provided funding only:

the Kaiser Family Foundation data on U.S. funding for HIV/AIDS, and FCAA *Report on HIV/AIDS Grantmaking by U.S. Philanthropy.*

Area of Health Tracked

Several health resource data collections focus exclusively on the resources going to HIV/AIDS: CRIS, SIDALAC National HIV/AIDS Accounts, Idasa AIDS Budget Unit reports, the Kaiser Family Foundation reports on U.S. and global funding for HIV/AIDS, and the FCAA *Report on HIV/AIDS Grantmaking by U.S. Philanthropy.* In addition, CRS, AiDA, PHR*plus* NHA Subanalysis, and the Resource Flows Database contain data on the resources going to both HIV/AIDS and reproductive health. The data in the WHO report on global tuberculosis control focus exclusively on tuberculosis, a disease for which CRS and AiDA also contain data. CRS and AiDA also contain some data on malaria activities, and PHR*plus* is currently preparing a malaria subanalysis.

Other areas of health that are tracked by the existing data collections include immunizations, physicians, hospital beds, and health related commodities. For example, the Immunization Financing Database and WDI both track expenditures on immunizations, and WDI also tracks the number of physicians and hospital beds in developing countries. The Database of Trade in Health Related Goods and Services in the Americas tracks imports and exports of health related goods or commodities, including pharmaceutical, medicinal chemical, and botanical products, and medical and surgical equipment and orthopedic appliances.

Resource Transaction Chain

The resource transaction chain describes the flow of health resources from (1) the entities that provide the resources (both cash and in-kind) to (2) those that receive the resources to (3) the goods and services acquired through the use of the resources and, finally, to (4) the target populations and/or beneficiaries actually receiving the goods and services. All of the health resource data collections in this inventory contain information on the resource providers (e.g., national governments, bilateral/multilateral donors, NGOs, development banks, private foundations, industry, private health insurance, and out-of-pocket spending). Several also provide information on the resource recipients—CRS, the Resource Flows Database, AiDA, the Kaiser Family Foundation reports on U.S. and global funding for HIV/AIDS, CRIS, Idasa, and NHA, National HIV/AIDS Accounts, and NHA subanalyses conducted by WHO, PHR*plus*, and SIDALAC. Few, however, provide information on the goods and services acquired with the funding provided—CRIS, the Immunization Financing Database, NHA, National HIV/AIDS Accounts, and NHA subanalyses (WHO, PHR*plus*, and SIDALAC). And even fewer provide information on the target population and/or beneficiaries actually receiving the resources—CRIS, NHA, National HIV/AIDS Accounts, and NHA subanalyses conducted by WHO, PHR*plus*, and SIDALAC.

External Resource Flows

No one health resource data collection contains data from all donors on all external resource flows. For example, CRS, which is the most extensive database on donor aid, contains no data on bilateral aid flows from non-DAC members (such as China) or on aid flows from the core budgets of NGOs. Other donor flows that are not captured by the existing data collections include donations from private foundations, charities, faith-based organizations, and pharmaceutical companies, as well as donations of medical devices and aid for building health care infrastructure (e.g., education and training).

Domestic Resource Flows

The current collections also do not provide complete information on the domestic resource flows of all developing countries. The WHO NHA database, for instance, contains the most extensive collection of information on health care expenditures, covering indicators for 192 of its member states, and yet it is not comprehensive and lacks critical detail. Data are also needed for expenditures that occur below the national levels of governments—that is, at the regional, district, and local levels. Idasa has conducted analyses of the HIV/AIDS budget in South Africa at the provincial level, but most of the other data collected on health resources provide information at the national level only. Information on private flows of health resources, including out-of-pocket spending, private insurance, private industry, NGOs, and NPISH, is not covered adequately. NHA do attempt to collect information on some of these private flows, but the data in these cases are incomplete. Moreover, data on technical cooperation (e.g., transfers of know-how and technologies) are difficult to track and generally are not reported. For example, even though OECD/DAC collects this information from DAC members in CRS, other data collectors do not have comparable information.

Data Quality and Harmonization

To be of the greatest use, data should be continuous over time and regularly checked for accuracy and reliability. The definitions, methods, and conventions used by the data collectors should be harmonized as much as possible to facilitate comparisons of data obtained by different organizations. While the NHA methodology has become more standardized, especially with the recent release of a new user's guide and training manual, other data collectors continue to use their parochial definitions, methods, and conventions, with the result that comparisons between data collections are very difficult.

"Cost" of Data Collection

At present, a constant tension seems to exist between the need for more timely, detailed, and complete data on health resources and the ability to get those data. The more comprehensive the data collection, the more it costs to undertake and the longer it takes to complete. For example, the process of preparing NHA is both laborious and time-consuming, requiring special teams trained in NHA methodology, substantial planning, and extensive data collection from the health sector, which means from ministries, donors, providers, private insurers, employers, pharmaceutical companies, and households. The NHA methodology has become more standardized, but the process still varies from country to country depending on the structure of the health system and the country's capacity to prepare NHA, not to mention the budget and the political context of the country. Simplifying the approach used to track health resources could improve the timeliness, quality, and quantity of data. In addition, attention needs to be paid to building and maintaining the data collection capacity of developing countries.

Linkage to Other Relevant Datasets

Information on other areas is lacking as well, including data on training and education, capacity building, and health services (e.g., health personnel, hospital beds). Additionally, data systems need to have linkages between them—for example, there should be linkages between NHA and donor expenditures by country. However, before there can be linkages, the data collectors' definitions, methods, and conventions will have to be harmonized.

Summary

The data collections described in this chapter (and for which more detail is provided in Appendices B and C) represent significant efforts on the part of numerous entities to track the health resource flows in developing countries. These collections are capable of offering valuable insight into the overall trends in donor aid and country-level resource flows. However, as noted above, there are significant gaps in both the data and the understanding of global health resource flows. The health resource data presently available provide a patchwork of information at different levels of aggregation and resolution and of varying quality and timeliness. As a result, the data, collectively, fall short of what is needed to best serve the many and diverse purposes and organizations.

Most of the data gathered on health resources focus exclusively either on donor aid or on country-level expenditures but not on the linkage between the two.[40] The few data collections that do encompass both donor aid and country-level expenditures tend to focus on a single disease rather than on general health. Because most of these data concentrate on a specific country, disease, or type of resource, the current health resource data collections do not provide a complete and accurate picture of the health resource flows to and within developing countries on a global basis. Also, as noted above, several data collections contain information that is already two years out of date when it is released. And finally, many current data collectors gather their information using laborious collection techniques that require extensive planning and specially trained data collection teams, all of which place a large burden on those who are to contribute the data.

To produce a current, comprehensive picture of the health resources available to developing countries, the existing data collections must be improved or a new, less burdensome approach must be developed. Any data system designed to collect current, comprehensive data on global health resource flows would have to (1) be designed for the express purpose of tracking global health resources, (2) contain the most current information available (preferably real-time data, whenever available), and (3) be fed directly from transactional sources in order to reduce (perhaps eliminate) the reporting burden on data contributors. The framework for such a health resource data system and a new approach for creating it are described in the next chapter.

---

[40] One exception is the ratio of external resources to total health expenditures that WHO reports in its *World Health Report* and on its Website. This information is obtained from country reports and triangulated with OECD DAC data.

CHAPTER THREE

A Global Health Resource Tracking System

A single health resource tracking system, if designed, configured, and populated properly, should be able to accommodate the data needs of all users worldwide—be they donors of health resources, recipients of health resources, or some other interested party. Such a data system would begin by identifying all health resources the moment they entered any one of the "streams" composing the worldwide flow of such resources, and would then follow them through all of their "handlers" and "transformations" to the point at which they were finally "provided." Specifically, a truly global health resource tracking system would be able to annually identify and assemble information set forth in the budgets of *all* countries (including developing countries) and private entities around the world that had to do with *all* planned activities designed to address any of the health care needs of a developing nation. This information would include both the amount of funds involved and a detailed description of the purpose(s) of the funding, and it would serve as the baseline for a truly global health resource tracking system.

As these planned activities were set into motion, the funds budgeted to pay for them would be tracked as they were converted into obligations and then into outlays/expenditures. Concomitantly, the transformation of these funds from plans into reality would be tracked and described in the global health resource tracking system, as would all of the "hands" through which these funds passed during this transformation. Consider the following example, in which a developed nation has budgeted funds for addressing global health needs via the health assistance program of an international organization. These funds would first be tracked from the developed nation to their receipt by the international organization. From there, they would be tracked as they were combined with similar funds from other countries and then used to pay the costs of transporting the vaccine that had been donated by a pharmaceutical company and the travel of volunteers to administer the vaccine to children in a specific developing nation. Once in the developing nation, this resource stream would have added to it the resources contributed directly by the developing nation: a government truck, driver, and petrol to transport the volunteers in country. The ideal health resource tracking system would seamlessly follow and integrate all of these cash and in-kind resource streams in real time without double-counting *and* without placing more than a minimal reporting burden on any of the entities involved. In short, a truly global health resource tracking system must

- Contain valid, detailed data (who, what, where, how much) on all of the health resources (cash and in-kind) provided last year (expenditures), provided this year (obligations), and to be provided next year (budgeted) to all developing countries by all public and private entities in virtually real time without double-counting any of the resources.

- Impose no more than a minimal burden on any public or private entity in terms of what is necessary to provide the information needed to populate the system.
- Readily harmonize with and connect to existing data systems of both countries and donors.
- Be easily accessible via the Web and flexibly searchable from every angle in a variety of languages.
- Enjoy broad ownership, official buy-in, and use, with long-term support from a diversified funding base.

While the core data in such a system would be freely available to all interested parties, some data could be maintained in one or more protected areas of the tracking system for access by special permission only. And finally, since information on health resource flows is rarely by itself sufficient to support the type of policy-relevant analysis needed to facilitate better decisionmaking, it will likely be important that the information in the global health resource tracking system be easily connected to such critical complementary data as general demographic information, population surveys, epidemiological studies, and various socioeconomic indicators. With proper planning and support, much, if not all, of this critical complementary information could be routinely maintained on the servers containing the global health resources tracking or on parallel servers.

What Data Are Essential?

Clearly, not all of the data we have just described for a truly global health resource tracking system are essential to a serviceable health resource tracking system. But it is not easy to identify which bits and pieces of these data are essential and which are expendable. Indeed, any determination of which data elements are to be considered truly essential in a basic health resource tracking system would likely depend on one's role in the provision of health resources to developing countries. For example, it is unlikely that the donors of health resources and the countries dealing directly with their citizens' health needs will focus on the same pieces of information when making their crucial decisions. Given this reality, it seems unwise to attempt to determine which data are absolutely needed in a basic health resource tracking system. A more productive approach might be to prioritize the data we have described as part of the global health resource tracking system according to the needs of such a system's users, and then to focus on where to start assembling these data.

Such an approach would begin with an inventory of all currently existing administrative systems from which one or more of the pieces of information could be obtained. Once this inventory were completed, its results would be mapped against the data elements contained in the global data system and a determination would be made as to where (and how) the missing data could be obtained and what level of priority should be given to obtaining them. With this information, a master plan could be created that (1) spells out which data would be available in a central health resource tracking system and when, and (2) describes how and when the gaps in the data could or would be filled.

Gaps in Currently Available Data

Even before making an inventory of all the health resource data that exist in some form somewhere, we know of specific gaps in the data that all interested parties would like to see filled. For example, there are gaps in the data detailing

- Past and current health budgets of all countries contributing health resources of any kind
- Past and current health spending of all resource providers (both public and private)
- In-kind donations of health resources (e.g., pharmaceuticals, training of personnel)
- Out-of-pocket spending on health care by citizens in developing countries
- Institutional capacity and level of training of personnel in developing countries
- In-country spending on and distribution of health resources
- The nature, extent, and impact of trade and tax subsidies involving health resources
- The effect of patents and other intellectual property on resource availability and flows.

This list is not exhaustive, but it illustrates the breadth of the gaps in the currently available data on health resources. It also shows that there are many places where one can begin to build the data system for tracking the health resources needed by and available to developing countries.

A Different Approach to Collecting Data

Many health resource tracking activities rely on information collected through surveys of government, nongovernmental organization (NGO), bank, foundation, organization, or corporate officials about the institutions for which they are responsible. While definitely of value, surveys have distinct limitations as data collection tools. First, surveys typically are unable to filter out the subjective perceptions of respondents. No matter how carefully the purpose, scope, and categories of a survey are described and defined in the survey instrument, the respondent's background, training, and professional experience will color his or her answers to the survey questions. When the survey involves a complex topic (e.g., global health resource flows), reasonable people will be especially likely to differ as to what the appropriate answer might be to any particular question. Second, surveys are intrusive in that they require the time and cooperation of respondents who will receive little, if any, benefit from their effort.

An alternative approach that avoids the problems of surveys is the use of "unobtrusive measures." Moreover, the most common type of unobtrusive measure is the running record that is created by a government or other entity as it conducts its routine business. And because the most common type of running record is a transactional record that memorializes an exchange of money, running records are ideally suited unobtrusive measures for tracking the flow of resources among various entities.

The RaDiUS Database at RAND, which annually tracks the tens of billions of dollars spent by the U.S. government on research and development (R&D), is the foremost example of a resource tracking system populated entirely with data *not* collected using surveys.

Instead, all data in the RaDiUS Database are regularly collected unobtrusively by piggy-backing on the existing records of the U.S. federal government. In both the United States and abroad, this pioneering use of unobtrusive measures to create a major resource tracking system is of interest to many who envision its potential application to a variety of challenges—including the tracking of health resources around the world. Unobtrusive measures and the RaDiUS Database are described in more detail in the following sections.

Unobtrusive Measures

In the 1960s, a quartet of noted social scientists formally introduced the world to the concept of unobtrusive measures in a book so titled. At that time, much like today, the vast majority of data collected about various topics was gathered via surveys using questionnaires or structured interviews. The scientists noted that this method is an intrusive way of collecting data that is "limited to those who are accessible and will cooperate, and the responses obtained are produced by dimensions of individual differences irrelevant to the topic at hand" (Webb et al., 1966, p. 1). They lamented the fact that few took advantage of the unobtrusive measures that exist in many places (such as the running records kept by governments), which might yield better information on a given subject than the intrusive method of collecting data using surveys. While not perfect, such unobtrusive measures have quite "different methodological weaknesses" than do surveys (Webb et al., 1966).

A decade ago, RAND, in cooperation with the National Science Foundation (NSF), began a project to identify and determine the potential usefulness of unobtrusive measures for tracking federal R&D funding and activities. This effort, which eventually became known as the RaDiUS (Research and Development in the United States) program, identified numerous pockets of data within the federal government that contained useful information on federal R&D funding and/or activities that were housed in offices throughout the U.S. government and, most importantly, were regularly updated and often had built-in self-validation mechanisms. The most visible of these pockets of data were the federal-level and agency-specific budgets of the U.S. government. Many of the pockets of data were available for internal agency use only, and some were formal agency-specific databases available to the general public only on a selective basis. Three were official governmentwide data systems available to the general public in some form. These three—the Federal Procurement Data System (FPDS), the Federal Assistance Awards Data System (FAADS), and the Catalog of Federal Domestic Assistance (CFDA)—were found to contain very valuable information on federal R&D funding, although none of them had been created specifically to do so.

The information gathered by the FPDS and FAADS are transactional records in that they record and document the details of the multitude of individual financial transactions carried out each year between the U.S. government and specific nongovernmental individuals and/or entities. The FPDS collects detailed information on every large contract (over $25,000) awarded by the federal government. The FAADS is the counterpart of the FPDS in that it collects detailed information on all "nonprocurement" financial awards made by the federal government to third parties (grants, cooperative agreements, loans, direct payments, etc). Every award in FAADS is linked to one of the programs listed in the CFDA, which is a compendium of all programs, projects, services, and other types of assistance provided to nonfederal entities by all agencies of the U.S. government. The CFDA is routinely used by nonfederal entities to determine which of the funds they receive each year come from the federal government.

By weaving the information in the FPDS, FAADS, and CFDA together, RAND found that the vast majority of federal R&D funding could be tracked without having to field any surveys. Clearly, the accuracy of this R&D funding information is unparalleled, as it is extracted from official government data systems (i.e., running records) that are monitored, maintained, and corrected whenever errors are noted. And all of these data can be obtained in virtually real time without imposing any additional reporting burdens on government officials or members of the private sector. In short, the RaDiUS Database shows that by piggybacking on the running records of governments and weaving the gathered information together to form a database, one is using unobtrusive measures—most especially, the transactional records of governments—as the source of critically needed data that are both more accurate and more timely than data collected via surveys.

Using Unobtrusive Measures to Track Health Resources

Every entity that provides health resources to developing countries maintains some sort of records of the amount of resources they provide each year and the identity of the recipients. In developed countries, international organizations, and NGOs that provide cash with which to purchase health resources in developing countries, these records are budgets and/or procurement and disbursement documents. In entities that provide in-kind health resources to developing countries (e.g., pharmaceuticals), these records are product distribution and/or shipping documents. Once received by developing countries, these resources, combined with resources provided by the developing countries themselves, can be tracked in-country using the internal disbursement and distribution documents maintained by the national, regional, and/or local governments, as well as by the international organizations and NGOs that are operating internally in these countries.

These "business" records that are routinely generated by governments, international organizations, corporations, and NGOs are the unobtrusive measures upon which a global health resource tracking system could, and indeed should, be based, for two reasons. First, such running records are of unparalleled accuracy and cost nothing to collect. Second, only by piggybacking on these running records to create a global health resource tracking system can the information in the system be virtually real time.

There are limitations to the use of unobtrusive measures, however. For example, accessing and linking data from large complex databases with disparate structures and formats can be quite challenging. This is especially true when different countries and organizations may have quite different ways of organizing and/or maintaining their records. In addition, such data are not always accurate, reliable, or valid—i.e., definitions of terms may change from year to year without being noted, and archival records can be subject to errors and changes in record-keeping procedures. And sometimes the data are altered for political reasons. However, it is possible to verify the accuracy of data obtained through unobtrusive measures by checking it against information obtained from other sources (i.e., triangulation).

There could be additional challenges involved in using unobtrusive measures, as well. Countries with few resources and little institutional capacity may not maintain centralized, electronic records of health resource flows. Still, in a significant number of countries with large populations as well as considerable health expenditures and needs (e.g., Brazil, South Africa, India), data systems are likely to be sufficiently advanced for the use of unobtrusive measures to be feasible. In addition, some entities, such as private corporations and foundations, may be unwilling to share some information that they regard as proprietary. However, information is usually more accessible from public entities (e.g., governments, international organizations, NGOs), many of which are required to publicly report financial data. Several other factors can also make the collection and comparison of data from different countries challenging, including different languages and currencies; diverse accounting practices, data collection procedures, and data gathering systems; and dissimilar structures of health care systems.

In short, while the creation and continuous updating of a global health resource tracking system using unobtrusive measures would not be trivial, it appears to be feasible on a technical level. The open question is whether it is feasible on a political level.

Users of a Global Health Resource Tracking System

The potential users of the truly global health resource tracking system described above include countries, international organizations, corporations, and NGOs. That is, when policy leaders and decisionmakers in any of these entities focus their substantive interests on global health resources, they will likely want to know

- What external entities are providing health resources to developing countries?
- How are these externally provided health resources allocated among developing countries?
- What health resources are developing countries providing internally?
- How are these internally provided health resources combined with externally provided health resources and distributed within the nation?
- How are health resources being used? How much is actually getting to the intended recipients?

Why they want answers to these questions and how they will use the information provided depend directly on the nature of their interest in global health resources. For example, those interested in providing or facilitating the provision of health resources (the donors) will want a slightly different set of information than will developing countries receiving health resources (the recipients).

Donors, be they countries, international organizations, corporations, or NGOs, want a health resource tracking system that tells them what other donors are providing to developing countries in the way of health resources so that they can determine the best way to help and can gauge whether their fellow donors are doing their fair share to address a global problem. They also want to be able to determine what differences the health resources they provide are making: Are the provided health resources replacing health resources that the recipients would and/or could otherwise provide themselves? Or are the provided health resources truly adding new capabilities/capacity to the health resources already available to the recipients (i.e., additionality). In short, donors want access to data that will help them effectively mobilize and target the health resources that they provide to developing countries.

Recipients, however, want information that allows them to account for all of the health resources they have at their disposal, both to demonstrate that they are providing whatever resources they can to address their nation's health problems and to ensure that they make effective use of the health resources they have. Recipients also need to be able to measure success (as well as defeat) in their battle against infectious diseases and other health care challenges: They want to detect a decline in hospital patient populations, document an increase in people vaccinated against some disease, etc. In short, recipients want access to data that tell them how they are doing in their struggle against all the health-related challenges they face.

Thus, although both donors and recipients of health resources will be active users of a truly global health resource tracking system, the two sectors are likely to tap slightly different portions of the system in order to obtain the information needed to guide the health-related decisions and activities that are of most direct concern to them.

CHAPTER FOUR

Conclusions

Governments, international organizations, for-profit corporations, and nonprofit organizations throughout the world regularly provide both cash and in-kind health resources to help address the health needs of developing countries. Currently, these health resources are not tracked on a global level and no information source exists to provide an overall picture of who is giving what resources to whom and for what purpose. As a result, policymakers in developing and developed countries alike have no ongoing access to comprehensive, accurate, timely data on the resources being devoted to health in developing countries. And without these data, none of the parties trying to address the health problems of developing countries has the empirical knowledge required to answer a variety of questions and to inform policy decisions about health resource mobilization and allocation, strategic planning, priority setting, monitoring and evaluation, advocacy, and general policymaking.

A number of entities are presently involved in significant efforts to track the flow of health resources to and/or within developing countries. Our inventory of these existing health resource data collections provides an in-depth analysis of the purpose, content, strengths, and limitations of these systems. In this chapter, we draw implications from our inventory of available data collections and our discussion of an "ideal" system as these shed light on the potential next steps involved in creating a comprehensive global health resource tracking system that will meet the needs of the global health community and address the limitations of current systems.

Gaps in Current Data Collection Efforts

As our inventory shows, many bilateral assistance agencies, multilateral and research/advocacy organizations, and developing country governments have mounted significant efforts to track health resource flows in developing countries. However, from a global perspective, these efforts are fragmented, and significant gaps remain in the substance of the data, which are also hampered by inaccuracy and a general lack of timeliness. Moreover, the data exist at many disparate levels of aggregation and resolution, and many of the data collections focus exclusively on either donor aid or country-level expenditures, with very few capturing data on both.

Our inventory identified several gaps in the current health resource data collections, including

- No one collection contains data from all donors of health resources

- Data on health resource flows are not available for all countries
- The data are of varying degrees of timeliness and quality
- The data collectors' definitions, methods, and conventions vary widely, making it difficult to compare and/or integrate different collections
- The data are not accessible to all potential users.

Using Current Health Resource Tracking Efforts

Despite these deficiencies, the current disparate collection of data on health resources provides the raw material with which a more comprehensive, unified data system could possibly be built—if only as a stop-gap measure. Specifically, many of the health resource data collections described in our inventory have significant strengths. These collections provide valuable information about overall trends in donor aid and financial flows within the health sectors of developing countries, and they contribute key input for advocacy, strategic planning, priority setting, monitoring and evaluation, and evidence-based policymaking. And at least some of these data collections are timely, high quality, and detailed. As a result, it might be possible to assemble some core information on global health resources in the near term by tapping these data collections and integrating and harmonizing their contents as much as possible. This is not a long-term solution to the challenge confronted, but it would buy some much needed time in which to explore options on how best to build a global system that tracks all health resources flowing to and within developing countries.

Next Steps: Developing Technical Specifications for a Comprehensive Global Health Resource Tracking System

Potentially, the next step toward developing a global health resource tracking system would be to convene an expert group to develop technical specifications for designing and implementing a new comprehensive strategy for collecting data. Some of the issues that these experts could address are: What new data are needed? What are the pros and cons of different approaches to collecting the data? What technological considerations enter into designing and implementing a global system? The points below illustrate key issues that an expert group would likely need to consider.

Additional Data

What data would a more comprehensive data system need to include? Clearly, any health resource tracking system would have to include much of the "core" data already being collected, albeit in improved form (e.g., more detailed using standardized definitions). But as we note in Chapter Three, some important data are not being collected at all: current (as well as past) health budgets of countries contributing health resources; current (as well as past) health spending of all resource providers; in-kind donations of health resources (pharmaceuticals, training of personnel, etc.); out-of-pocket spending on health care by citizens in developing countries; institutional capacity and level of training of personnel in developing countries; in-country spending on and distribution of health resources; trade and tax subsidies involving health resources; and the impact of patents and other intellectual property on resource availability and flows. Clearly, the group of experts designing a new health resource tracking system would weigh the value of including these data in a new system, as well as other data not yet identified.

A Different Approach to Collecting Data

We note in Chapter Three that many current data collection efforts rely on surveys of government, nongovernmental organization (NGO), bank, foundation, organization, or corporate officials about the institutions for which they are responsible, and that the two major drawbacks to this approach are maintaining up-to-date information and filtering out the subjective impressions of respondents. An alternative way to track health resources is to rely more extensively on information collected for other purposes, such as the budgeting, procurement, and disbursement data in administrative records. These records, which are "unobtrusive measures" (in contrast to "intrusive" surveys), could be used either as the base for a new global health resource tracking system or to improve existing data collections. Piggybacking on these records to create a global health resource tracking system could provide accurate, virtually real-time data for the information system. The use of unobtrusive measures is one way to solve the needs of the international community for a global health resource tracking system.

In conclusion, better data and better resource tracking systems are needed to give policymakers and those providing aid to developing countries better and more reliable information upon which to base their decisions. Providing the needed data will require a comprehensive strategy for data collection that can accurately show the resources being brought to bear by all parties—developing countries, developed countries, international organizations, corporations, and private nonprofit organizations—to combat disease and improve health in developing countries. Creating such a strategy will require a fundamental rethinking of how health resources can be tracked on a global basis. Furthermore, given the general lack of complete, accurate, up-to-date, and detailed data and the complexity of the problem, any solution is likely to require a great deal of cooperation and commitment on the part of the providers and the recipients of health resources alike.

Participants in Technical Consultation on Health Resource Tracking Held by the Center for Global Development and RAND, May 10–11, 2004

Name	Organization	Title
Sono Aibe	The David and Lucile Packard Foundation	Senior Program Manager
Ross Anthony	RAND Corporation	Associate Director for Global Health
Julia Benn (participated via teleconference)	OECD/DAC (Organisation for Economic Co-operation and Development/Development Assistance Committee)	Administrator, Statistics and Monitoring Division, Development Co-operation Directorate (DCD)
Peter Berman	Harvard School of Public Health	Professor of Population & International Health Economics; Director of International Health Systems Program
Stan Bernstein	Millennium Project	Sexual and Reproductive Health Policy Adviser
Stefano M. Bertozzi	Instituto Nacional de Salud Publica	Director, Health Economics
Karen Cavanaugh	USAID (United States Agency for International Development)	Health Systems Management Analyst
Don Creighton	Pfizer, Inc. Corporate Affairs	Manager, Global Policy/Corporate Policy & Strategic Management
Paul De Lay	UNAIDS (Joint United Nations Programme on HIV/AIDS)	Director, Monitoring and Evaluation
Jacqueline Eckhardt-Gerritsen	NIDI (Netherlands Interdisciplinary Demographic Institute)	Project Leader, Resource Flows Project
Elisa Eiseman	RAND Corporation	Policy Analyst
Sally Ethelston	Population Action International	Vice President for Communications
Donna Fossum	RAND Corporation	Program Manager and Senior Policy Analyst
Tamara Fox	William and Flora Hewlett Foundation	Program Officer, Population Programs
Joel Friedman	Center on Budget & Policy Priorities	Senior Fellow
Amparo Gordillo-Tobar	PAHO (Pan American Health Organization)	Consultant on Health Economics and Financing
Pablo Gottret	World Bank	Senior Health Financing Economist
Brian Hammond (participated via teleconference)	OECD/DAC	Head, Statistics and Monitoring Division, DCD
Alison Hickey	Idasa (Institute for Democracy in South Africa)	Manager, AIDS Budget Unit, Budget Information Service

Name	Organization	Title
John Howe III	Project HOPE	President & CEO
Jose-Antonio Izazola-Licea	SIDALAC (Regional AIDS Initiative for Latin America & Caribbean)	Executive Coordinator
Jennifer Kates	Kaiser Family Foundation	Director, HIV Policy
Kei Kawabata	WHO (World Health Organization)	Coordinator of Resource Flows, Expenditures, and Risk Protection Team
Patience Kuruneri	WHO	Senior Adviser, Roll Back Malaria Partnership Secretariat
Bill Leinweber	Research America	Vice President
Ruth Levine	CGD (Center for Global Development)	Senior Fellow and Director of Programs
Maureen Lewis	CGD	Senior Fellow
Eric Lief	Independent consultant	
Bill McGreevey	The Futures Group International	Director, Development Economics
Catherine Michaud	Harvard Center for Population and Development Studies	Senior Research Associate
Emiko Naka	GFATM (Global Fund to Fight AIDS, Tuberculosis, and Malaria)	
Mead Over	World Bank	Senior Economist, Development Research Group
Rudolphe Petras	OECD/DAC	Administrator, Statistics and Monitoring Division
Ravi P. Rannan-Eliya	Health Policy Programme, Institute of Policy Studies	Associate Fellow
Blair Sachs	Bill & Melinda Gates Foundation	Program Officer, Global Health Policy & Finance
Russ Scarato	USAID	Health Economist
Nina Schwalbe	Open Society Institute	Director, Public Health Programs
Barbara Seligman	USAID	Senior Policy Advisor, Bureau of Global Health
David Sevier	MAPA Ventures	Principal
James Sherry	Global Health Council	Vice President, Policy, Research & Advocacy
Anil Soni	Friends of the Global Fund	
Sergio Spinaci	WHO	Executive Secretary, Coordination of Macroeconomic & Health Support Unit, Sustainable Development & Health Environments
Todd Summers	Progressive Health Partners	President
Ron Waldman	Millennium Project	Head of Maternal and Child Health Task Force; Clinical Professor of Epidemiology
Veronica Walford	Institute for Health Sector Development (UK)	Director
Joseph C. Whitehill	Congressional Budget Office, U.S. Congress	Senior Analyst, International Development
Virginia Yee	World Bank	Director, Accessible Information on Development Activities (AiDA) Development Gateway Foundation

APPENDIX B
Inventory of Health Resource Data Collections

Table B.1
Inventory of Health Resource Data Collections

	Data on Donor Aid					Data on Donor Aid and Country-Level Expenditures/Activities	
	CRS (Creditor Reporting System) Database on Aid Activities	AiDA (Accessible Information on Development Activities)	Report on HIV/AIDS Grantmaking by U.S. Philanthropy	U.S. Government Funding for HIV/AIDS in Resource Poor Settings	Global Funding for HIV/AIDS in Resource Poor Settings	Resource Flows Database	Global Tuberculosis Control: Surveillance, Planning, Financing
Primary organization collecting data	OECD/DAC	Development Gateway Foundation	FCAA	Kaiser Family Foundation	Kaiser Family Foundation	UNFPA/UNAIDS/NIDI	WHO
Years data collected	1967–2004[1]	1970–2004	2000–2002	1986–2004	1996–2004	1997–2002[5]	2002–2004
How often data collected/updated	quarterly	monthly, quarterly, annually[3]	annually	annually	annually	annually; biennially[6]	annually
Year latest data available	2003	2004	2002	2005	varies by sector	2002[5]	2002 (expenditures); 2003 (budget)[8]
Publicly available	yes	yes	yes	yes	yes	yes[7]	yes
Data available about countries in following regions							
East Asia and Pacific	X	X			X	X	X
Europe and Central Asia	X	X			X	X	X
Latin America and the Caribbean	X	X			X	X	X
Middle East and North Africa	X	X			X	X	X
South Asia	X	X			X	X	X
Sub-Saharan Africa	X	X			X	X	X
United States and Canada	X	X	X	X	X	X	
Other	OECD/DAC member countries[2]			PEPFAR countries[4]			22 HBCs[9]

Table B.1 (continued)

	Data on Donor Aid					Data on Donor Aid and Country-Level Expenditures/Activities	
	CRS (Creditor Reporting System) Database on Aid Activities	AiDA (Accessible Information on Development Activities)	Report on HIV/AIDS Grantmaking by U.S. Philanthropy	U.S. Government Funding for HIV/AIDS in Resource Poor Settings	Global Funding for HIV/AIDS in Resource Poor Settings	Resource Flows Database	Global Tuberculosis Control: Surveillance, Planning, Financing
Source of data							
Survey/questionnaire	X		X			X	X
Transactional data (direct feed)	X	X					
National reports				X		X	
International reports					X		
Other (describe specifically)	Excel files	Websites of development organizations	Foundation Center data	appropriations legislation; legislative report language; U.S. agency estimates; other official government budget reports	UNAIDS; FCAA; other studies	OECD/DAC; case/thematic studies	NTPs, GFATM, WHO CHOICE Website, and other costing studies
Partner organizations	World Bank	Bellanet, OECD/DAC, World Bank					
Data collection status							
Primary data	X		X	X	X	X	X
Secondary data		X	X		X	X	X
Granularity of data							
Aggregate/summarized			X	X	X		
Detailed (specify)	project	project				project	line item

Table B.1 (continued)

	Data on Donor Aid					Data on Donor Aid and Country-Level Expenditures/Activities	
	CRS (Creditor Reporting System) Database on Aid Activities	AiDA (Accessible Information on Development Activities)	Report on HIV/AIDS Grantmaking by U.S. Philanthropy	U.S. Government Funding for HIV/AIDS in Resource Poor Settings	Global Funding for HIV/AIDS in Resource Poor Settings	Resource Flows Database	Global Tuberculosis Control: Surveillance, Planning, Financing
Responding/reporting entities							
Country/government				X	X	X	X
Bilateral donors	X	X			X	X	X
Multilateral donors	X	X			X	X	
International NGOs		X			X	X	
Development banks	X	X			X	X	
Private foundations		X	X		X	X	
National NGOs		X			X	X	
Industry/corporate foundations			X		X		
Other	DAC member		public charities			national consultants	National TB Control Program
Type of funding reported							
Budget				X	X		X
Obligations/commitments	X	X	X	X	X		X
Disbursements/expenditures/outlays	X	X			X	X	X
Other							funding gaps; future resource requirements
Type of dollars reported							
National currency unit	X	X				X	
US $		X	X	X	X	X	X
International $ (PPPs)		X					
Other							

Table B.1 (continued)

	Data on Donor Aid					Data on Donor Aid and Country-Level Expenditures/Activities	
	CRS (Creditor Reporting System) Database on Aid Activities	AiDA (Accessible Information on Development Activities)	Report on HIV/AIDS Grantmaking by U.S. Philanthropy	U.S. Government Funding for HIV/AIDS in Resource Poor Settings	Global Funding for HIV/AIDS in Resource Poor Settings	Resource Flows Database	Global Tuberculosis Control: Surveillance, Planning, Financing
Resource transaction chain							
Providers of resources							
Country/government					X	X	X
Bilateral donors	X	X			X	X	X
Multilateral donors	X	X			X	X	X
International/national NGOs		X		X	X	X	
Development banks	X	X	X		X	X	X
Private foundations			X		X	X	
Industry/corporate foundations							
Private health insurance							
Patients (out-of-pocket spending)							
Other	DAC member		public charities				GFATM
Recipients of resources	X	X		X	X	X	
Acquired goods and services							
Target population/beneficiaries							
Other							
Area of health tracked							
Health (non-disease specific)							
HIV/AIDS	X	X	X	X	X	X	
TB	X	X					X
Malaria	X	X					
Population/reproductive health	X	X				X	
Other	sector/purpose codes	X				basic research, data, and population and development policy analysis	

Table B.1 (continued)

	OECD Health Data	WHO National Health Accounts	Data on Country-Level Expenditures/Activities (National Health Accounts, National HIV/AIDS Accounts, and Other Disease-Specific Subanalyses)		
			Health Accounts/ National Health Accounts	PHR*plus* National Health Accounts	National HIV/AIDS Accounts
Primary organization collecting data	OECD	WHO	PAHO	PHR*plus*/ Abt Associates	SIDALAC
Years data collected	1960–2003[10]	1995–2002[12]	1990–2001	1995–2001	1995–2002
How often data collected/updated	annually	annually	country dependent	country dependent	country dependent
Year latest data available	2002[10]	2001[12]	2001	2001	2002
Publicly available	yes	yes	yes	yes	yes
Data available about countries in following regions					
East Asia and Pacific	X	X		X	
Europe and Central Asia	X	X		X	
Latin America and the Caribbean	X	X	X	X	X
Middle East and North Africa		X		X	
South Asia		X		X	
Sub-Saharan Africa		X	X	X	X
United States and Canada	X	X	X	X	
Other	OECD member countries[11]				

Table B.1 (continued)

	Data on Country-Level Expenditures/Activities (National Health Accounts, National HIV/AIDS Accounts, and Other Disease-Specific Subanalyses)				
	OECD Health Data	WHO National Health Accounts	Health Accounts/National Health Accounts	PHR*plus* National Health Accounts	National HIV/AIDS Accounts
Source of data					
Survey/questionnaire	X	X	X	X	X
Transactional data (direct feed)					
National reports	X	X	X	X	X
International reports	X	X	X	X	X
Other (describe specifically)	NHA; HA; NA; OECD estimates[13]	household surveys, EUROSTAT, OECD, IMF, UN and regional commissions, UNPOP, Carricom, World Bank, development banks, regional WHO offices, EIU	household surveys	household surveys	household surveys
Partner organizations		OECD, World Bank, USAID, SIDA	IDB, World Bank, USAID	WHO, World Bank, PAHO, SIDA, UNICEF, and others	
Data collection status					
Primary data	X	X	X	X	X
Secondary data	X	X	X	X	X
Granularity of data					
Aggregate/summarized	X	X[14]	X		
Detailed (specify)				line item	line item

Table B.1 (continued)

	Data on Country-Level Expenditures/Activities (National Health Accounts, National HIV/AIDS Accounts, and Other Disease-Specific Subanalyses)				
	OECD Health Data	WHO National Health Accounts	Health Accounts/National Health Accounts	PHRplus National Health Accounts	National HIV/AIDS Accounts
Responding/reporting entities					
Country/government	X	X	X	X	X
Bilateral donors		X		X	X
Multilateral donors		X		X	X
International NGOs		X			X
Development banks		X		X	X
Private foundations				X	X
National NGOs		X		X	X
Industry/corporate foundations		X		X	X
Other			households; private insurance	insurance companies; hospitals; large employers	
Type of funding reported					
Budget					
Obligations/commitments					
Disbursements/expenditures/outlays	X	X	X	X	X
Other					
Type of dollars reported					
National currency unit	X	X	X	X	X
US $		X	X	X	X
International $ (PPPs)		X	X	X	
Other					

Table B.1 (continued)

	Data on Country-Level Expenditures/Activities (National Health Accounts, National HIV/AIDS Accounts, and Other Disease-Specific Subanalyses)				
	OECD Health Data	WHO National Health Accounts	Health Accounts/ National Health Accounts	PHR*plus* National Health Accounts	National HIV/AIDS Accounts
Resource transaction chain					
Providers of resources					
Country/government	X	X	X	X	X
Bilateral donors	X	X	X	X	X
Multilateral donors	X	X	X	X	X
International/national NGOs	X	X	X	X	X
Development banks	X	X	X	X	X
Private foundations	X	X	X	X	
Industry/corporate foundations	X			X	
Private health insurance	X	X	X	X	X
Patients (out-of-pocket spending)	X	X	X	X	X
Other		social health insurance; parastatals; private firms			
Recipients of resources	X	X	X	X	X
Acquired goods and services	X	X		X	X
Target population/beneficiaries	X	X		X	X
Other					
Area of health tracked					
Health (non-disease specific)	X	X	X	X	
HIV/AIDS		X		X	X
TB					
Malaria				X	
Population/reproductive health				X	
Other					

Table B.1 (continued)

			Data on Country-Level Expenditures/Activities (Other)			
	World Development Indicators	**NHExp Database**	**Database of Trade in Health Related Goods and Services in the Americas**	**Idasa Budget Information Service Budget Briefs and Reports**	**Immunization Financing Database[17]**	**Country Response Information System[20]**
Primary organization collecting data	World Bank	PAHO	PAHO	Idasa	GAVI	UNAIDS
Years data collected	1960-2003[15]	1980– 2001	1994-2000	1995-2004	1999-2004[18]	2003-2004
How often data collected/updated	annually	annually	annually	annually[16]	annually	country dependent
Year latest data available	2003[15]	2001	2000	2003/04 budget; 2005/06 MTEF	2003	2003
Publicly available	yes	yes	yes	yes	yes	yes
Data available about countries in following regions						
East Asia and Pacific	X				X	X
Europe and Central Asia	X				X	X
Latin America and the Caribbean	X	X	X		X	X
Middle East and North Africa	X				X	X
South Asia	X				X	X
Sub-Saharan Africa	X					X
United States and Canada	X	X	X	X		X
Other				South Africa	GAVI eligible countries[19]	

Table B.1 (continued)

	Data on Country-Level Expenditures/Activities (Other)					
	World Development Indicators	NHExp Database	Database of Trade in Health Related Goods and Services in the Americas	Idasa Budget Information Service Budget Briefs and Reports	Immunization Financing Database[17]	Country Response Information System[20]
Source of data						
Survey/questionnaire				X		
Transactional data (direct feed)						X
National reports	X	X		X		
International reports	X	X				
Other (describe specifically)	varies by responding/ reporting entity	household surveys	DATAINTAL 3.1	interviews	Financial Sustainability Plan	
Partner organizations		WHO	WHO		various[21]	X
Data collection status						
Primary data	X	X	X	X	X	
Secondary data	X	X		X		
Granularity of data						
Aggregate/summarized	X	X	X			
Detailed (specify)				program; line item	cost category[22]	project

Table B.1 (continued)

			Data on Country-Level Expenditures/Activities (Other)			
	World Development Indicators	NHExp Database	Database of Trade in Health Related Goods and Services in the Americas	Idasa Budget Information Service Budget Briefs	Immunization Financing Database[17]	Country Response Information System[20]
Responding/reporting entities						
Country/government	X	X	X	X	X	X
Bilateral donors						
Multilateral donors						
International NGOs						
Development banks						
Private foundations						
National NGOs						
Industry/corporate foundations						
Other	central banks; customs services		international organizations		GAVI eligible countries	
Type of funding reported						
Budget				X	X	
Obligations/commitments						
Disbursements/expenditures/outlays	X	X		X	X	X
Other			value of imports and exports	MTEF	future resource requirements, financing, and gaps	
Type of dollars reported						
National currency unit	X	X	X	X	X	X
US $						
International $ (PPPs)						
Other						

Table B.1 (continued)

	Data on Country-Level Expenditures/Activities (Other)					
	World Development Indicators	NHExp Database	Database of Trade in Health Related Goods and Services in the Americas	Idasa Budget Information Service Budget Briefs and Reports	Immunization Financing Database[17]	Country Response Information System Project Resource Tracking Database[20]
Resource transaction chain						
Providers of resources						
Country/government	X	X	X	X	X	X
Bilateral donors					X	X
Multilateral donors					X	X
International/national NGOs				X	X	X
Development banks					X	X
Private foundations					X	X
Industry/corporate foundations						X
Private health insurance	X	X				
Patients (out-of-pocket spending)	X	X				
Other		NPISH	international trade in health related commodities		Vaccine Fund	
Recipients of resources						
Acquired goods and services			X	X	X	X
Target population/beneficiaries						X
Other			imports/exports			X
Area of health tracked						
Health (non-disease specific)	X	X				
HIV/AIDS				X		X
TB				X		
Malaria						
Population/reproductive health						
Other	immunizations; physicians; hospital beds		health related commodities		immunizations	

Key
BIS = Budget Information Service
DAC = Development Assistance Committee
EIU = Economist Intelligence Unit
EUROSTAT = Statistical Office of the European Communities
FCAA = Funders Concerned About AIDS
GAVI = Global Alliance for Vaccines and Immunization
GFATM = Global Fund to Fight AIDS, Tuberculosis, and Malaria
HA = Health Accounts
HBC = High-Burden Countries (for tuberculosis)
HIV/AIDS = Human Immunodeficiency Virus/Acquired Immunodeficiency Syndrome
IDB = Inter-American Development Bank
IMF = International Monetary Fund
MTEF = Medium Term Expenditure Framework
NA = National Accounts
NHA = National Health Accounts
NHExp = National Health Care Expenditure
NIDI = Netherlands Interdisciplinary Demographic Institute
NPISH = Nonprofit Institutions Serving Households
NTP = National Tuberculosis Control Program
OECD = Organisation for Economic Co-operation and Development
PAHO = Pan American Health Organization
PEPFAR = President's Emergency Plan for AIDS Relief
PHR*plus* = Partners for Health Reform*plus*
SIDA = Swedish International Development Cooperation Agency
SIDALAC = Regional AIDS Initiative for Latin America and the Caribbean
TB = Tuberculosis
UN = United Nations
UNAIDS = Joint United Nations Programme on HIV/AIDS
UNFPA = United Nations Population Fund
UNPOP = United Nations Population Division
USAID = United States Agency for International Development
WHO = World Health Organization
WHO CHOICE = WHO CHOosing Interventions that are Cost-Effective

Footnotes
[1] Data from 1973 onward are available online.
[2] The OECD/DAC members are Australia, Austria, Belgium, Canada, Denmark, Finland, France, Germany, Greece, Ireland, Italy, Japan, Luxembourg, Netherlands, New Zealand, Norway, Portugal, Spain, Sweden, Switzerland, United Kingdom, United States, and the Commission of the European Communities.
[3] Information is updated monthly, quarterly, or annually depending on the participating organization. The date of the last update is displayed in each record.
[4] The 15 priority PEPFAR countries are Botswana, Côte d'Ivoire, Ethiopia, Guyana, Haiti, Kenya, Mozambique, Namibia, Nigeria, Rwanda, South Africa, Tanzania, Uganda, Vietnam, and Zambia.

[5]Estimates for 2003 expenditures are also available.

[6]Donor data are collected annually; domestic data are collected biennially.

[7]Disaggregated/project level data are proprietary and not publicly available; aggregate data are available in UNFPA's *Financial Resource Flows for Population Activities* report.

[8]Beginning in 2004, WHO is asking for budget data for both the current year (year t) and the previous year (year t–1).

[9]The HBCs for TB are Afghanistan, Bangladesh, Brazil, Cambodia, China, Democratic Republic of Congo, Ethiopia, India, Indonesia, Kenya, Mozambique, Myanmar, Nigeria, Pakistan, Philippines, Russian Federation, South Africa, Thailand, Uganda, United Republic of Tanzania, Vietnam, and Zimbabwe.

[10]Selected Secretariat estimates are available for 2003.

[11]The OECD member countries are Australia, Austria, Belgium, Canada, Czech Republic, Denmark, Finland, France, Germany, Greece, Hungary, Iceland, Ireland, Italy, Japan, Korea, Luxembourg, Mexico, Netherlands, New Zealand, Norway, Poland, Portugal, Slovak Republic, Spain, Sweden, Switzerland, Turkey, United Kingdom, and United States.

[12]WHO has data for 1950 to 2002, but only the 1995–2001 data are publicly available.

[13]The data sources for the OECD Health Data fall into four groups: (1) NHA (following SHA methodology); (2) locally produced health accounts (HA); (3) National Accounts; (4) estimates made by the OECD Secretariat.

[14]For some countries, information is available at the level of line items, providers, and function; however, the level of detail varies depending on the availability of the data from each country.

[15]2003 data for selected indicators only.

[16]Data on the HIV/AIDS budget in South Africa are produced annually. Data for a multicountry study on Argentina, Chile, Ecuador, Mexico, Namibia, Nicaragua, Mozambique, Kenya, and South Africa were collected for the first time in 2004. A second phase of this multicountry study will involve more countries in Sub-Saharan Africa and will be conducted over the next two and one-half years.

[17]The data contained in the Immunization Financing Database are derived from the Financial Sustainability Plans (FSPs) countries submit to GAVI at the midpoint of their funding from the Vaccine Fund.

[18]Data are only available starting in 2000 for some countries.

[19]The GAVI eligible countries are governments in the 75 poorest countries (GNI below US$1000).

[20]The information in the table is for the Project Resource Tracking (PRT) database, one of three databases making up the Country Response Information System. PRT was released in August 2004; training and support activities will be provided over the next year to maximize its use at the country level.

[21]Abt-Associates (PHR*plus*), World Bank, PAHO, UNICEF, Children's Vaccine Program, Vaccine Fund, and Center for Global Development.

[22]Cost category includes: (1) recurrent costs, which are vaccines, injection supplies, personnel, transport, cold chain maintenance, building overheads, training, social mobilization, IEC, monitoring and surveillance; and (2) capital costs, which are vehicles, cold chain equipment, and buildings.

Inventory of Health Resource Data Collections—Detailed Descriptions

Data on Donor Aid

Creditor Reporting System (CRS)—Database on Aid Activities

Description

The Organisation for Economic Co-operation and Development (OECD) Development Assistance Committee (DAC) is primarily responsible for carrying out OECD's work related to cooperation with developing countries. DAC collects and publishes statistics on aid and other resource flows to developing countries and countries in transition, based principally on reports from DAC members.[1] The work of DAC is supported by the Development Co-operation Directorate, (DCD), which is often referred to as the "DAC Secretariat" because of this key function.

The Creditor Reporting System (CRS), an online database developed and maintained by DAC, presents the official statistics for the financial flows of official development assistance (ODA) and official aid (OA) of DAC members.[2] CRS provides textual and numerical information on individual transactions (e.g., specific projects). The data are collected for the specific purpose of providing information to DAC members so that they can provide better aid, and DAC members are the primary clients of the database. The objective of DAC and the CRS database is to collect and publish timely information and comprehensive statistics of official and private flows of aid to recipient countries.

DAC also maintains a companion database to the CRS, the DAC Database on Annual Aggregates, which provides aggregate data on the volume, origin, and types of aid and other resource flows to over 180 recipients (developing countries and countries in transition).

---

[1] DAC members are those members of the OECD that give the most aid; they provide more than 90 percent of all aid to developing countries and countries in transition. DAC member nations are Australia, Austria, Belgium, Canada, Denmark, Finland, France, Germany, Greece, Ireland, Italy, Japan, Luxembourg, Netherlands, New Zealand, Norway, Portugal, Spain, Sweden, Switzerland, United Kingdom, United States, and the Commission of the European Communities (OECD/DAC, http://www.oecd.org/document/38/0,2340,en_2649_33721_1893350_1_1_1_1,00.html).

[2] Official development assistance (ODA) is aid, in the form of grants or loans, given to countries and territories on Part I of the DAC List of Aid Recipients ("traditional" developing countries). Aid to the "more advanced" eastern European and developing countries (those on Part II of the list) is recorded separately as official aid (OA). The DAC List of Aid Recipients is used to help measure and classify aid and other resource flows originating in DAC countries. It is available online at http://www.oecd.org/document/45/0,2340,en_2649_34469_2093101_1_1_1_1,00.html.

It includes each recipient's intake of ODA, OA, and other official and private funding from DAC members, multilateral agencies, and other donors. The DAC Database measures the flows of aid and other financial resources to aid recipients, broken down by major category of expenditure. The data cover aid loans and grants, other official flows, private market transactions, and assistance from nongovernmental organizations (NGOs) to each recipient country and recipient countries combined. The DAC Database provides aggregate information on aid flows, and CRS provides detailed information at the project level.

Data Collection

CRS provides a set of basic data on financial flows of ODA and OA that can be used to analyze where aid goes, what purposes it serves, and what policies it supports. Data are available at the level of individual projects or in aggregate tabular form. CRS contains the title and a short description of the projects, but no abstracts or detailed project descriptions are available online. Long descriptions are stored in an internal database at DAC and can be made available upon special request.

Data are provided via questionnaires submitted by all DAC members. Reporting to DAC by non-DAC donors is done on a voluntary basis. The database also includes loan transactions by World Bank, Inter-American Development Bank (IDB), African Development Bank, and International Fund for Agricultural Development.

CRS reporting is quarterly, and the database is updated quarterly. Ideally, data for the previous year should be available by April of the current year (e.g., 2003 data would be available in CRS by April 2004). In reality, however, data for the previous year are not available until the end of the current year.

Funding amounts in CRS are commitments (obligations)—i.e., the face value of the activity on the date a grant or loan agreement is signed with the recipient. Total commitments per year comprise new undertakings entered into in the year in question (regardless of when disbursements are expected) and additions to agreements made in earlier years. Cancellations and reductions of earlier years' agreements are not taken into account.[3]

Data on disbursements each year are available at the activity level for approximately 70 to 80 percent of donors. Disbursement data are available online, but they are not as complete as the data on commitments. DAC has always requested these data, but they were unavailable until ten years ago, when it became possible to link accounting (i.e., disbursements) to project management systems (i.e., commitments).

DAC does not currently collect the following data:

- *European Commission (EC) data.* Some aid-extending agencies of the Commission of the European Communities do not report their activities to the CRS.
- *Data on multilaterals.* Multilaterals are not required to report to DAC and are difficult to obtain data from. World Bank and other regional banks, United Nations Children's Fund (UNICEF), and United Nations Population Fund (UNFPA) do submit information to DAC. United Nations Development Programme (UNDP),

---

[3] User's Guide to the online Aid Activity database, http://www.oecd.org/document/50/0,2340,en_2649_34469_14987506_1_1_1_1,00.html.

however, provides only estimates, and some smaller agencies, which are less important than UNDP in terms of donation amounts, provide no data.[4]

- *Private flows.* CRS does not cover money collected by NGOs themselves (private
  flows). It does, however, cover aid "through" NGOs, such as co-financing (joint financing) between NGOs and governments; DAC member (donor) contributions to
  the core budget of an NGO, and NGOs working as implementing agencies for DAC
  donors.
- *Domestic finances.* In-country resource flows are difficult to follow. This is mostly
  done through case studies—e.g., those of UNFPA/Netherlands Interdisciplinary
  Demographic Institute (NIDI).

CRS also does not include information about

- Bilateral aid flows from non-DAC members (such as China)
- Aid flows from the core budgets of NGOs
- Foreign direct investment, unguaranteed bank lending, portfolio investment
- Contributions by DAC members to multilateral agencies[5]
- Loans made out of funds held in the recipient country.

Accessible Information on Development Activities (AiDA)

Description
Accessible Information on Development Activities, or AiDA, as it is better known, is an online database containing a catalog of information on development activities found on the
Websites of development organizations. Participating organizations share information on
planned, current, and completed projects and programs that they fund, execute, or implement. AiDA aims to meet the demand for timely and reliable information about who is doing what in various locations and with what results.

AiDA is an activity of the Development Gateway Foundation, a nonprofit organization whose mission is to increase knowledge sharing, improve public sector transparency and
government efficiency, enhance the effectiveness of development assistance, and build local
capacity. Bellanet, OECD/DAC, and World Bank are jointly implementing this initiative.[6]
AiDA builds on the work of the International Network for Development Information Exchange (INDIX) and the International Development Mark-up Language (IDML) initiative
and organizations that are participating in this project.

Data Collection
AiDA contains a subset of information that participating organizations make available on
their Websites. It uses IDML to integrate information from multiple sources to enable search
and retrieval from a common interface in order to give users a single, consolidated report that

---

[4] Many multilaterals have their own internal classification systems and do not use the same codes as DAC uses to classify
activities (e.g., the UN's codes do not necessarily match up with DAC's).

[5] Contributions by DAC members to multilateral agencies are not available in CRS but are available in aggregate form in
the DAC Database on Annual Aggregates.

[6] AiDA, http://aida.developmentgateway.org/AidaAbout.doc.

includes development activities of different agencies. Users can get information by different criteria, such as country, sector or topic, funding organization, or status of activity. Information is provided at an activity level; an activity may be a strategic objective, program, project, or subproject.

Organizations participating in AiDA include donors, implementing agencies, and content aggregators. They share information on planned, current, and completed projects and programs that are available on their Websites or internal information systems. Data in AiDA do not replace official data found on the Websites of participating organizations. AiDA contains a subset of information and refers users to the source sites for further information when it is available.

The scope of information and the frequency of updates in AiDA vary by source. Information is updated monthly, quarterly, or annually depending on the schedules of the participating organizations.

The following organizations and networks are sharing information through AiDA:[7]

Primary sources of donor information:

- Inter-American Development Bank (IDB)
- International Development Research Centre (IDRC) Development Research Information System
- International Monetary Fund (IMF)
- John D. and Catherine T. MacArthur Foundation
- Natural Resources Information System (NARSIS)
- United Kingdom Department of Foreign International Development (DFID)
- United Nations Capital Development Fund (UNCDF)
- United Nations Population Fund (UNFPA)
- United States Agency for International Development (USAID)
- World Bank Projects.

Aggregators of donor information:

- Creditor Reporting System (CRS), with information from 23 members and major multilateral organizations.

Aggregators of information by region, country, or theme:

- Fundacion Acceso
- Current Agricultural Research Information System (CARIS)
- Electronic Networking for Rural Asia/Pacific Projects (ENRAP)
- El Salvador Country Gateway
- Global Knowledge Activity Information Management System (GKAIMS)
- India Development Information Network (INDEV)
- International Telecommunications Union (ITU)
- Program and Project Information System on Education (PRISME)

---

[7] http://aida.developmentgateway.org/AidaSourcesDesc.do.

- Web-based Information System for Agriculture and Sustainable Rural Development.

Information from the following sources is located in the AiDA historical repository:

- Development Activity Information (DAI)
- Development Cooperation Analysis System (DCAS)
- Mines Action Canada
- Open Society Internet Program.

AiDA is the largest single source of integrated information on development activities, but it is not yet comprehensive or up to date. It contains a total of 480,571 records— 430,743 in the current sources section, and 49,828 in the AiDA historical repository. The coverage and quality of the information are improving as more organizations participate in AiDA.

In addition, organizations report on activities at different levels, ranging from strategic objectives, programs, projects, subprojects, technical assistance, and study grants. AiDA does not have detailed enough information to make it possible to distinguish between these different levels.

Report on HIV/AIDS Grantmaking by U.S. Philanthropy

Description

Funders Concerned About AIDS (FCAA), organized in 1987, is an affinity group[8] of grantmakers whose mission is to mobilize "philanthropic leadership and resources, domestically and internationally, to eradicate the HIV/AIDS pandemic and to address its social and economic consequences."[9] FCAA has a core constituency of over 2,600 individuals, including private foundations, corporate grantmakers and giving programs, community and family foundations, United Ways, other charitable organizations, key government and public policy officials, UN officials, and media contacts.[10] FCAA is not a grantmaking organization and does not provide direct assistance to HIV/AIDS organizations or others interested in identifying or seeking potential grants from private funders.

FCAA has put out a series of publications on HIV/AIDS-related grantmaking by all sectors of U.S. philanthropy. The most recent FCAA publication, *Report on HIV/AIDS Grantmaking by U.S. Philanthropy*, includes lists of the top 50 HIV/AIDS grantmakers for the years 2001 and 2002, data for 2001 and 2002 about U.S.-based HIV/AIDS grantmaking, research on the corporate response to HIV/AIDS, and information about the regional and international distribution of private U.S.-based HIV/AIDS grants (Funders Concerned About AIDS, 2003). This report serves both as a practical tool for grantmakers in developing and sustaining their HIV/AIDS efforts and as a resource for those outside of philanthropy

---

[8] Affinity groups are groups composed primarily of grantmakers. Group activities must be open to any Council on Foundations member who would like to participate. The services and programs offered must be primarily for the benefit of grantmakers (Council on Foundations, http://www.cof.org/files/Documents/Networking/Affinity%20Groups/AGNcriteria-application4-2004.doc).

[9] http://www.fcaaids.org/about/.

[10] http://www.fcaaids.org/about/.

who want to better understand the critical role grantmakers play in the response to the pandemic and to work more effectively with grantmakers in enhancing all types of resources flowing to HIV/AIDS initiatives.

Data Collection

The 2003 FCAA report summarizes HIV-related grant commitments for 2001 and 2002 from all sectors of U.S. philanthropy, including private, family, and community foundations, public charities, and corporate grantmaking programs (Funders Concerned About AIDS, 2003). The report also contains information about the regional and international distribution of private, U.S.-based HIV/AIDS grants. In addition, it has information on in-kind donations that the corporate sector contributed to HIV/AIDS, such as resources in communications and marketing, logistics and distribution, human resource and application of information technology; and workplace programs such as nondiscriminatory policies, awareness and prevention (including distribution of condoms), and access to care, support, and treatment.

FCAA tracks and reports on grant commitments in each calendar year rather than on grant spending in a given year (Funders Concerned About AIDS, 2003). Multiyear grants are counted fully in the year when they are initially committed. This is consistent with the data collection methods of the Foundation Center; the Funders Network on Population, Reproductive Health, and Rights; and several other affinity groups (Funders Concerned About AIDS, 2003).

Information for the FCAA report came from a survey distributed in July 2003 to 78 grantmakers that requested specific information about their HIV/AIDS-related funding allocations in 2001 and 2002. When information was not available directly from these grantmakers, FCAA conducted additional research and collected additional HIV/AIDS grantmaking data from the Foundation Center and other sources to produce an unduplicated total set of 407 grantmakers. Data collected by FCAA surveys and other research methods were also compared with Foundation Center statistics for 2001 and 2002. The 2002 data in the *Report on HIV/AIDS Grantmaking by U.S. Philanthropy* are less comprehensive and final than the 2001 data (Funders Concerned About AIDS, 2003).

FCAA does not track the activities of faith-based organizations, governments, and international institutions involved in HIV-related grantmaking. However, FCAA is working in partnership with other organizations to support a broad coalition effort aimed at mapping the full multisectoral response to HIV/AIDS (Funders Concerned About AIDS, 2003). These partners include the Joint United Nations Program on HIV/AIDS (UNAIDS), World Bank, Henry J. Kaiser Family Foundation, Global Business Coalition on HIV/AIDS, and European HIV/AIDS Funders Network.

U.S. and Global Funding for HIV/AIDS in Developing Countries

Description

The Henry J. Kaiser Family Foundation is a nonprofit, private operating foundation that focuses on the major health care issues facing the United States.[11] The Kaiser Family Foundation HIV/AIDS Policy Program focuses on the HIV/AIDS epidemic both in the United

---

[11] Henry J. Kaiser Family Foundation, http://www.kff.org/about/index.cfm.

States and globally. The program's work in HIV/AIDS policy includes analysis and monitoring of

- Key epidemic trends
- Global and domestic spending on HIV/AIDS
- Major programs that provide prevention, care, and treatment to people at risk for and living with HIV/AIDS
- Public opinion about HIV/AIDS
- The impact of the epidemic on those populations and regions of the United States and the world that have been most affected, including young people, women, and minority communities.[12]

The Kaiser Family Foundation HIV/AIDS Policy Program performs primary research on U.S. funding and gathers secondary data on global funding for HIV/AIDS in developing countries. It produces a series of policy briefs, fact sheets, and other publications on domestic and global spending on HIV/AIDS. This work is ongoing and is updated on a regular basis. The most recent work in this area includes two policy briefs: (1) "U.S. Government Funding for Global HIV/AIDS Through FY 2005" (Kates and Summers, 2004), which provides detailed data on U.S. government funding for the global HIV/AIDS epidemic through FY 2004 and for the FY 2005 budget request; and (2) "Global Funding for HIV/AIDS in Resource Poor Settings" (Summers and Kates, 2003a), which summarizes data on the range of resources currently directed to address the HIV/AIDS epidemic in developing countries, including bilateral and multilateral support from donor governments, private sector support (i.e., support from corporations, foundations, and NGOs), and domestic funding by governments of developing countries.

Data Collection

The methods that the Kaiser Family Foundation uses for data collection and the data it makes available on global HIV/AIDS funding are not the same for U.S. government funding and for other funding (e.g., other major bilateral donors, affected country governments, and foundations). We thus describe them separately here.

U.S. Government Funding for HIV/AIDS in Resource Poor Settings. The Kaiser Family Foundation has data on U.S. government funding of HIV/AIDS in resource poor settings that extend from the beginning of the U.S. government role in global HIV/AIDS funding in FY 1986 through the President's budget proposal for FY 2005. The policy brief "U.S. Government Funding for Global HIV/AIDS Through FY 2005" (Kates and Summers, 2004) presents an overview chart of federal HIV/AIDS spending for FY 1986 through FY 2005 broken down by whether the funding was for bilateral programs; contributions to the Global Fund to Fight AIDS, Tuberculosis, and Malaria (GFATM); or for international research.

Data on U.S. government global HIV/AIDS funding are available at the program level for the federal departments/agencies responsible for the most U.S. international HIV/AIDS activities:

---

[12] From the Henry J. Kaiser Family Foundation, http://www.kff.org/about/hivpolicy.cfm.

- United States Agency for International Development (USAID)
- Department of State
- Centers for Disease Control and Prevention (CDC)
- National Institutes of Health (NIH)
- Department of Defense (DOD)
- Department of Labor (DOL)
- Department of Agriculture (USDA).

Information about other federal agencies that provide funding for global HIV/AIDS activities but do not receive funding targeted by Congress for this purpose is not available. These agencies are the Health Resources and Services Administration (HRSA), which provides support for treatment and care; the U.S. Census Bureau, which supports international epidemiology estimates; and the Peace Corps, which provides volunteers in many highly affected countries (Summers and Kates, 2003b).

Information is available about U.S. contributions to multilateral organizations, including GFATM and UNAIDS. General support from the United States to the UN, which indirectly provides funds to a wide variety of UN organizations involved in HIV/AIDS activities—such as the World Health Organization (WHO), UNICEF, and UNDP—is not included in the estimates of total U.S. global HIV/AIDS funding, because the United States does not designate specific amounts for HIV/AIDS activities by these organizations within its general contributions (Summers and Kates, 2003b). Information about the President's Emergency Plan for AIDS Relief (PEPFAR)—a five-year, $15 billion initiative to address HIV/AIDS, tuberculosis, and malaria in 15 of the hardest hit countries in the world—is also available.[13]

Most of the data on U.S. government funding of HIV/AIDS represent funds specifically designated (earmarked) for global HIV/AIDS programs or initiatives in accordance with either bill text or final report language of appropriations legislation (Kates and Summers, 2004).[14] These data are presented as appropriations by agency, year, and program. Data on NIH and CDC funding of international HIV/AIDS research are presented as self-reported expenditures of past funding and estimates of future funding (Kates and Summers, 2004).[15] The data are from a variety of primary sources, including congressional appropriations legislation, federal budget documents, reports and estimates from government agencies, and analyses by the U.S. Congressional Research Service (Summers and Kates, 2003a).

Disaggregated information about how U.S. funding for global HIV/AIDS activities is used—including for research, for prevention, or for care, treatment, and support—is not available, the reasons being that programs have become increasingly integrated and that most U.S. agencies do not publicly report their funding levels according to these broad categories (Kates and Summers, 2004).

---

[13] The 15 priority PEPFAR countries are Botswana, Côte d'Ivoire, Ethiopia, Guyana, Haiti, Kenya, Mozambique, Namibia, Nigeria, Rwanda, South Africa, Tanzania, Uganda, Vietnam, and Zambia.

[14] Appropriations legislation sets funding levels both through specific references included in the actual text of bills and through "report language" from the written reports developed by the various congressional appropriations committees (Summers and Kates, 2003a).

[15] HIV/AIDS research is typically excluded from estimates of global need or overall spending that are prepared by UNAIDS and others, but it is included in U.S. government calculations of its support for global HIV/AIDS efforts.

Other Global Funding for HIV/AIDS in Resource Poor Settings. The most recent Kaiser Family Foundation policy brief on this subject, "Global Funding for HIV/AIDS in Resource Poor Settings" (Summers and Kates, 2003a) contains the estimated funding for 2003 by donor governments, governments of affected countries, multilateral organizations, and private sector donors—i.e., foundations, corporations, and NGOs. (Previous reports covered funding for 1996 through 2001.) It also contains estimates of current and future funding needs for addressing HIV/AIDS in developing countries for 2002 through 2007. It does not include estimates of individual and household spending in affected countries.

Funding levels are either reported as "budgeted" amounts or "actual spending." Budgeted amounts represent final appropriations by government donors and final commitments by private sector donors (Summers and Kates, 2003a). Actual spending represents disbursements or outlays, but some governments also include within actual spending the obligation of budgeted funds through legal agreements, contracts, or purchase orders (Summers and Kates, 2003a).

The data on funding by governments other than the United States are primarily provided by UNAIDS, which maintains a database to track allocations of funding for global HIV/AIDS by source and use (Summers and Kates, 2003a).[16] The UNAIDS data are based on data provided by collaborations with a variety of external partners, including UNFPA and NIDI on the Resources Flows Project, and members of the Global Resource Tracking Consortium for AIDS. (For a more detailed description of the Resource Flows Project, see section below on Resource Flows Database.)

The data on country-level spending are UNAIDS estimates of HIV/AIDS and sexually transmitted disease (STD) project expenditures by national governments of developing countries (Summers and Kates, 2003a). However, it is difficult to get timely, accurate, and comparable data on domestic spending on HIV/AIDS activities, because health budgets in many affected countries do not isolate HIV/AIDS from other health and social service categories, and many countries lack the government infrastructure needed to maintain detailed budgetary information on HIV/AIDS spending (Summers and Kates, 2003a).

The data on HIV/AIDS funding by foundations, corporations, and NGOs come primarily from two sources: FCAA, for estimates of HIV/AIDS-related grantmaking by foundations and corporations, and UNAIDS, for estimates of actual disbursements by foundations and large international NGOs (Summers and Kates, 2003a). Funding for HIV/AIDS by foundations and corporations is difficult to track because grantmaking is often reported under broad and nonstandardized categories not specifically identified as HIV/AIDS, such as reproductive health and community-based health care. In addition, single-year funding is difficult to estimate because foundations and corporations frequently make multiyear grant commitments (Summers and Kates, 2003a). Attempting to estimate HIV/AIDS-related contributions by large, international NGOs is also difficult, in this case because no tracking system exists to capture their funding (Summers and Kates, 2003a).

Other challenges and limitations to gathering and analyzing information on global funding for HIV/AIDS include the following (Summer and Kates, 2003a):

---

[16] The UNAIDS data for the Kaiser Family Foundation report were provided through publicly available documents and directly through a collaborative agreement with the Kaiser Family Foundation (Summers and Kates, 2003a).

- There is no uniform reporting system, and data are collected through a variety of mechanisms by many different organizations.
- Donors typically report expenditures with at least a one-year delay, making it difficult to provide timely data.
- HIV/AIDS funding is often integrated into broader categories, such as reproductive health and sexually transmitted diseases.
- Distinguishing budgeted funding levels from actual amounts disbursed is difficult and subject to interpretation, particularly when funds flow through multiple entities before reaching direct service providers or beneficiaries. For example, countries making contributions to the GFATM transmit their funds to its trustee (World Bank), which transfers monies to grantees that may then be used to fund subgrantees.
- There is typically a difference between budgeted funding levels and actual amounts disbursed, particularly with large donors. The variances, which can be quite large, are usually attributable either to delays in spending by donors as newly funded programs build to capacity or to the reservation of funds to fulfill multiyear contracts.

Data on Donor Aid and Country-Level Data

Resource Flows Database

Description

The United Nations Population Fund (UNFPA) has collected data on and reported on flows of international financial assistance to population activities since 1980. It began also collecting data on domestic resource expenditures in developing countries at the request of the Commission on Population and Development following the International Conference on Population and Development (ICPD) held in Cairo in 1994 (United Nations Population Fund, 2003). In a report entitled *Financial Resource Flows for Population Activities in 2002* (United Nations Population Fund, 2004),[17] UNFPA provides information on international assistance from 1992 to 2002 and domestic resource flows to population activities from 1997 to 2001. The report focuses on the flow of funds from donors through bilateral, multilateral, and nongovernmental channels for population assistance to developing countries and countries in transition. It also includes grants and loans from development banks for population activities in developing countries. Expenditures made by national governments and NGOs in developing countries and countries in transition are also summarized in the report.

The Netherlands Interdisciplinary Demographic Institute (NIDI), a research institute of the Royal Netherlands Academy of Arts and Sciences engaged in the scientific study of population, has been under contract to UNFPA since 1997 to collect data for the resource flows report. Working with UNFPA, NIDI created a Resource Flows Database of both donor and domestic expenditures on population activities. NIDI also evaluates and analyzes the data in collaboration with UNFPA. In 1999, the Joint United Nations Programme on HIV/AIDS (UNAIDS) joined the UNFPA/NIDI collaboration.

The purpose of the UNFPA/UNAIDS/NIDI collaboration, called the Resource Flows Project, is to establish a refined annual data collection, monitoring, and information

---

[17] This is the 16th edition of a report previously published under the title *Global Population Assistance Report*.

dissemination system on global financial flows for population activities in developing countries and countries in transition. The Resource Flows Database includes expenditure data on "population activities" in four categories: family planning services; basic reproductive health services; STD and HIV/AIDS activities; and basic research, data, and population and development policy analysis. The category "STD and HIV/AIDS activities" has four subcategories: STDs, HIV/AIDS prevention, HIV/AIDS care and treatment, and HIV/AIDS support/ social mitigation. The definition of *population activities* used by UNFPA/UNAIDS/NIDI covers the "costed population package" classification system outlined in paragraph 13.14 of the 1994 ICPD Programme of Action and the key targets set out in the United Nations General Assembly Special Session (UNGASS) Declaration of Commitment on HIV/AIDS.[18]

Data Collection

The Resource Flows Project collects and reports data on international population assistance (i.e., international donors) and domestic (i.e., national government and NGO) expenditures for population activities in developing countries and countries in transition. Data are collected through mail surveys/questionnaires, case studies, and the OECD/DAC database. The mail surveys consist of two independent parts: (1) an annual donor questionnaire distributed to approximately 180 donors (OECD/DAC countries, foundations, multilateral organizations and agencies, international NGOs, development banks, and universities and research institutions); and (2) a biennial domestic questionnaire distributed to government departments, national NGOs, and national consultants in developing countries and countries in transition.[19] To avoid double-counting, the data are collected at the project level but reported at an aggregate level.

In addition, the Resource Flows Project has conducted 15 country case studies to supplement the information gathered by the surveys. These case studies have been carried out in Brazil, China, Egypt, Ethiopia, India, Indonesia, Iran, Nigeria, Pakistan, Peru, Poland, Senegal, South Africa, Tanzania, and Thailand. They measure the financial resource flows for population activities within developing countries and describe the system of health sector financing and policy for population activities.

Data collected in the surveys and case studies are analyzed and published in

- The annual *Financial Resource Flows for Population Activities* report (e.g., United Nations Population Fund, 2003). (These reports are also available on the UNFPA Website, www.unfpa.org.)
- The *Report of the Secretary-General on the Flow of Financial Resources for Assisting in the Implementation of the Programme of Action of the International Conference on Population and Development* (e.g., United Nations, 2004), presented annually to the Commission on Population and Development.
- Case study reports.

---

[18] NIDI, http://www.nidi.nl/resflows/faqs.html.

[19] Beginning in 2003, data on domestic expenditures will be collected from a set of 61 core countries, which are developing countries and countries in transition that represent 80 percent of the total population of these regions, 90 percent of previously reported expenditures, and a fair balance in regional representation, as well as priority countries from an HIV/AIDS perspective. The other, noncore countries will be sampled every other year on a rotating basis. Core and noncore countries will be surveyed in alternate years, so all countries will have been surveyed over a four year period: core countries in 2004, a sample of noncore countries in 2005, core countries again in 2006, and the remaining noncore countries in 2007.

Information on the resource flows can also be found on the NIDI Website at www.nidi.nl/resflows.

The Resource Flows Database is not available online. All data gathered for the database are treated as confidential and remain the property of UNFPA, while data for HIV/AIDS expenditures are jointly the property of UNFPA and UNAIDS.

The Resource Flows Project does not collect data on expenditures by the private sector—i.e., private insurance, para-state organizations, private enterprises, out-of-pocket spending.

It is difficult to collect expenditures made at lower administrative levels (e.g., at regional and local levels). It is also increasingly difficult to estimate population expenditures when they are included as part of integrated programs and sector-wide approach (SWAp) programs. Another challenge is to institutionalize the data collection process in developing countries and countries in transition and to ensure its sustainability at the country level.

There is also the issue of obtaining timely data. Information is collected for the previous fiscal year, but because of the time needed for all respondents to report their expenditures and the data to be cleared, two years pass before the figures are released and the report is published (e.g., UNFPA's 2003 report is for expenditure data from 2001, year t–2). In 2003, NIDI conducted a pilot exercise to produce real-time (year t) estimates for donor assistance and domestic government expenditures for population activities for donors and developing countries/countries in transition. The need for more current data by UNFPA and UNAIDS has prompted NIDI to begin collecting year t estimations and year t+1 projections from 2004 onward.

Global Tuberculosis Control: Surveillance, Planning, Financing

Description

In March 2004, WHO released its eighth annual report on global tuberculosis control, *Global Tuberculosis Control: Surveillance, Planning, Financing* (World Health Organization, 2004a). The purpose of this series of annual reports is to chart progress in global tuberculosis control and progress in implementing DOTS (directly observed treatment, short-course), the strategy promoted by WHO and recommended internationally to control tuberculosis. The report contains data on the notification of tuberculosis cases and treatment outcomes from all national tuberculosis control programs that have reported to WHO. It also contains an analysis of plans, budgets, expenditures, and constraints on DOTS expansion for the 22 high-burden countries (HBCs) for tuberculosis.[20]

In 1991, the World Health Assembly ratified the following targets for global tuberculosis control by 2000: (1) to successfully treat 85 percent of detected smear-positive tuberculosis cases, and (2) to detect 70 percent of all smear-positive cases. Since these targets were not reached by the end of 2000, the target year has been reset to 2005. WHO's reports on global tuberculosis control provide eight consecutive years of data with which to assess pro-

---

[20] The HBCs for tuberculosis are Afghanistan, Bangladesh, Brazil, Cambodia, China, Democratic Republic of Congo, Ethiopia, India, Indonesia, Kenya, Mozambique, Myanmar, Nigeria, Pakistan, Philippines, Russian Federation, South Africa, Thailand, Uganda, United Republic of Tanzania, Vietnam, and Zimbabwe.

gress toward the 2005 global targets for case detection (70 percent) and treatment success (85 percent).

Data Collection

Beginning in 2002, the annual report on global tuberculosis control included financial analyses. The 2002 report presents annual financial requirements and funding gaps in the 22 HBCs for 2002 and for the period 2001–2005, based on five-year plans and costing studies. The 2003 report analyzes the funding requirements, funding sources, and funding gaps for the 22 HBCs for calendar year 2003 and includes revised estimates of funding gaps for planning period 2001–2005. The 2004 report (World Health Organization, 2004a) presents more-detailed data, including

- Total and per-patient National Tuberculosis Control Program (NTP) budgets and tuberculosis control costs, and funding sources and gaps related to these budgets and costs for HBCs in FY 2003.
- Total and per-patient NTP expenditures and tuberculosis control costs, and funding for these expenditures and costs for HBCs in FY 2002.
- Estimates of the total resources required to meet global targets for case detection and cure for HBCs in FYs 2004 and 2005.
- NTP budgets and funding gaps for other countries in FY 2003.

During 2003, a standard form for reporting surveillance and financial data was sent to 210 countries via WHO regional offices to request information about policy and practice in tuberculosis control, about the number and types of tuberculosis cases notified in 2002, and about the outcomes of treatment and retreatment for smear-positive cases registered in 2001 (World Health Organization, 2004a). It also asked for information about NTP budgets, expenditures, and funding sources, and about the way in which the general health infrastructure is used for tuberculosis control. NTP managers were asked to complete two tables, one about the NTP budget for FY 2003 and the funding and funding gaps related to that budget, and the other about NTP expenditures and the source of funds for those expenditures for FY 2002. Data from GFATM proposals, WHO CHOICE (CHOosing Interventions that are Cost-Effective) estimates of the costs of bed days and outpatient visits, and published and unpublished costing studies were also used. Costing guidelines developed for the Disease Control Priorities in Developing Countries Project (DCPP) were used to identify the purchasing power parity exchange rates.

NTP managers in the 22 HBCs were also asked, via a separate questionnaire and interviews, to summarize plans for tuberculosis control from 2003 onward, focusing on activities to improve political commitment, expand access to DOTS, strengthen diagnosis, improve treatment outcomes, ensure adequate staffing, and improve program monitoring and supervision (World Health Organization, 2004a). They were asked about collaborative tuberculosis/HIV activities, the management of drug resistance, and the development of partnerships, and to identify major constraints to reaching tuberculosis control targets (World Health Organization, 2004a).

A total of 201 countries reported to WHO on their strategies for tuberculosis control and on tuberculosis case notifications and/or treatment outcomes (World Health Organization, 2004a). Financial data were received from 123 countries, 77 (of which 17 were HBCs) providing complete data on 2003 budgets, and 74 (of which 15 were HBCs) providing complete, disaggregated expenditures for 2002 (World Health Organization, 2004a).[21]

Since the financial analysis for tuberculosis control began in 2002, WHO has continued to identify new areas to track. For example, WHO would like to track annual budget and expenditures for multi-drug-resistant tuberculosis and HIV-associated tuberculosis, and has added questions to the survey for the 2005 report to address this.

Information on individual grants is not available, because information is obtained only on "total grants." It is thus impossible to look at trends in grants from particular donors and to determine who the major donors are. For the 2005 report, NTP managers will be asked to complete a separate column on the tables for funds from GFATM, since it is a major donor to the HBCs.

Contributions given to the health sector as sectorwide grants or loans are not reported because it is difficult to separate out the amount specifically used for tuberculosis. These types of funds are usually reflected as government contributions because such disease-specific financing makes it difficult to determine where the funds originally came from.

Data on Country-Level Expenditures/Activities: National Health Accounts, National HIV/AIDS Accounts, and Other Disease-Specific Subanalyses

General Description

National Health Accounts (NHA) are an internationally accepted methodology used to determine a nation's total health expenditure patterns, including public, private, and donor spending (Partners for Health Reform*plus*, 2003a). NHA address four basic sets of questions: where do resources come from, where do they go, what kinds of services and goods do they purchase, and whom do they benefit (World Health Organization, 2002)? NHA attempt to answer these questions by showing the flow of financing from a source of funding to a particular use, to a user of that expenditure, or to beneficiaries, following a standard classification of health expenditure (World Health Organization, 2002). Basically, NHA show where the money comes from and where the money goes.

NHA were implemented in a number of middle- and low-income countries in the mid- to late 1990s. To date, approximately 70 countries around the world have conducted NHA, and more than 50 NHA have been conducted in low- and middle-income countries (Partners for Health Reform*plus*, 2003b). However, many countries have conducted only one study, with no repeat studies in subsequent years. Only one-third of the countries conducting NHA currently do so on a regular, sustained basis (Partners for Health Reform*plus*, 2002). Some countries that have been conducting NHA for a number of years—Mexico, Philippines, Bolivia, Nicaragua, Guatemala, and El Salvador—now have series of over five years' worth of data. Other countries—Morocco, Egypt, Jordan, Uganda, Kenya, and Zambia—also have multiple years' worth of data. Tracking health accounts over time allows trends in public and private spending on health to be monitored and analyzed.

NHA are designed to be comprehensive, recurrent, standardized, and comparable measures of expenditures on health care. They allow countries to visualize national expendi-

---

[21] Although financial data have been requested from the United States and Canada since 2003, there are no financial data available for these two countries.

tures on health care and provide policymakers with information on the distribution of health funds within the system. NHA can help policymakers in determining the health care system's level of efficiency and identifying areas of under- or overspending.[22] NHA can provide policymakers with useful information about the strengths and weaknesses of the health system, possible strategies for improving the efficiency and equity of health spending and government action in the sector, and the effects of policy changes on public and private spending patterns.[23] In addition, NHA allow the performance of one country's health system to be compared to those of others (Partners for Health Reform*plus*, 2002). NHA have been designed to be straightforward and easily understood by policymakers, including those without a background in economics (Partners for Health Reform*plus*, 2003a).

Several organizations are actively involved in the development, collection, dissemination, and analysis of NHA. OECD has been involved in the development of health accounts in its member states for over 30 years. More recently, WHO, the Pan American Health Organization (PAHO), and Partners for Health Reform*plus* (PHR*plus*) have been actively involved in conducting NHA in developing countries. WHO, PAHO, and PHR*plus* work collaboratively on the implementation of NHA, along with a number of other partners: World Bank, Swedish International Development Cooperation Agency (SIDA), Belgian Cooperation, Asian Development Bank, IDB, Norwegian Agency for Development Cooperation (NORAD), European Union (EU), and others.

The flexibility of the NHA framework also allows for the analysis of data on targeted populations or disease-specific activities, such as health expenditures related to child health or HIV/AIDS (Partners for Health Reform*plus*, 2003b). HIV/AIDS expenditures have been tracked using National HIV/AIDS Accounts in Latin America and the Caribbean with the support of the Regional AIDS Initiative for Latin America and the Caribbean (SIDALAC).[24] PHR*plus* has assisted countries in East, Central, and Southern Africa in conducting NHA subanalyses to track expenditures on HIV/AIDS, malaria, and reproductive health. WHO is also currently using NHA methodology to measure disease-specific expenditures. National HIV/AIDS Accounts and NHA subanalysis are important sources of information for evidence-based decisionmaking, but they are not simplistic exercises. Allocation of expenditures to specific disease groups often requires application of various estimation techniques, particularly in countries adopting integrated service delivery models.

NHA have their origins in the System of National Accounts (SNA). NHA and SNA share conceptual and methodological characteristics, but they evolved separately and are used for different purposes. SNA track factors of production and types of goods and services produced in the context of a nation's economy as a whole, whereas NHA track the flows of resources and expenditures among and between the various actors in the health system (World Health Organization, World Bank, and United States Agency for International Development, 2003). SNA are the responsibility of a country's national income accounts office; NHA are the responsibility of other agencies, especially ministries of health (Rannan-Eliya, Berman, and Somanathan, 1997).

---

[22] LAC (Latin American and Caribbean) Health Accounts, http://www.lachealthaccounts.org/en/keytopic.php?topic=33.

[23] LAC Health Accounts, http://www.lachealthaccounts.org/en/keytopic.php?topic=36.

[24] National HIV/AIDS Accounts are based on NHA methodology but are not necessarily a subanalysis of NHA. In the majority of countries that have conducted them, National HIV/AIDS Accounts are stand-alone exercises. SIDALAC has developed National HIV/AIDS Accounts in all 22 countries in which it has worked.

SNA are a standardized system of statistical analysis that provides a comprehensive and consistent picture of a country's entire economy (Organisation for Economic Co-operation and Development, 2000). They are built on decades of international consensus building and are internationally comparable and internally consistent (Rannan-Eliya, Berman, and Somanathan, 1997). SNA are established in line with international accounting standards, as detailed in the *System of National Accounts 1993*, a joint publication of Eurostat (the Statistical Office of the European Communities), IMF, OECD, United Nations Statistics Division, and World Bank (Commission of the European Communities et al., 1993). This publication contains recommendations on constructing "functionally-oriented satellite accounts," which are designed to support analysis of expenditures on a specific purpose, including health satellite accounts (World Health Organization, 2003). These health satellite accounts have the same objectives as NHA do, while maintaining an explicit linkage to the central SNA framework (Hjortsberg, 2001).

NHA describe the flow of resources specifically within the health sector. The methodology used for the WHO, PHR*plus*, and PAHO NHA and the methodology used for the OECD SHA embody most of the principles of the *System of National Accounts 1993*, but there are a number of differences (World Health Organization, 2002).[25] The most fundamental difference is that NHA focus on the flows of resources and expenditures between different institutional elements within a health care system, whereas SNA health satellite accounts show links between the health sector and the macroeconomy (Rannan-Eliya, Berman, and Somanathan, 1997). In addition, NHA have greater flexibility than SNA do in the use of data sources (Rannan-Eliya, Berman, and Somanathan, 1997).

The NHA approach is not yet standardized—methodologies and definitions differ from country to country. Several instruction manuals have been developed in an effort to standardize and simplify the NHA process:

- *A System of Health Accounts.* In May 2000, the OECD published the manual *A System of Health Accounts* (SHA) to improve the quality of international comparisons of data on health expenditures. This manual contains guidelines for reporting health expenditure according to an international standard. (Organisation for Economic Co-operation and Development, 2000.)

- *Guide to Producing National Health Accounts.* In 2003, WHO, World Bank, and USAID jointly published their *Guide to Producing National Health Accounts—With Special Application to Low-Income and Middle-Income Countries*. The guide provides conceptual and practical information about NHA to assist countries in implementing NHA to measure their national health expenditures. OECD's *A System of Health Accounts* served as the basis for this guide. (World Health Organization, World Bank, and United States Agency for International Development, 2003.)

- *National Health Accounts Training Manual.* In December 2003, PHR*plus* published the *National Health Accounts Training Manual* (Partners for Health Reform*plus*, 2003a). The manual is a "tool kit" for NHA trainers; it contains lectures, PowerPoint presentations, interactive exercises, and supplemental reading. It closely follows the

---

[25] For a detailed discussion of the similarities and differences in NHA and SNA, see the relevant sections in Organisation for Economic Co-operation and Development, 2000, Chs. 1 and 8; Hjortsberg, 2001, Ch. 3; and World Health Organization, World Bank, and United States Agency for International Development, 2003, Ch. 1.

methodology presented in the 2003 guide published by WHO, World Bank, and USAID (see directly above).

The 2003 guide developed by WHO, World Bank, and USAID represents an effort to harmonize and standardize the different approaches for producing NHA. However, some countries have not adopted the methodology presented in the guide. For example, three OECD member countries—Finland, New Zealand, and Poland—continue to use "locally produced health accounts" methodologies for determining health expenditures, and these differ from and vary in their degree of compatibility with NHA and SHA.[26] In addition, although more and more countries collect health expenditure data, only a limited number have produced full national health accounts (World Health Organization, 2004b).

NHA track total expenditures on health, which encompass all expenditures for activities whose primary purpose is to restore, improve, and maintain health for the nation and for individuals (Partners for Health Reform*plus*, 2003b). Health expenditures are commonly defined as all expenditures for prevention, promotion, rehabilitation, and care; population activities; nutrition; and emergency programs for the specific objective of improving or maintaining health. Health includes the health of individuals as well as of populations (Hjortsberg, 2001). Total expenditures on health are a combination of both public outlays and private outlays on health, as follows (World Health Organization, 2004b):

- *Public outlays on health.* The outlays earmarked for the enhancement of the health status of population segments and/or the distribution of medical care goods and services among population segments by
  — Central/federal, state/provincial/regional, and local/municipal authorities.
  — Extrabudgetary agencies and social security schemes, which include purchases of health goods and services by schemes that are compulsory and under governmental control.
  — External resources (mainly grants and credits with high grant components to governments). Grants to NGOs are accounted for as private expenditure but, in practice, are not always easily separated from public grants.
- *Private outlays on health.* The sum of the following:
  —Prepaid plans and risk-pooling arrangements, including private, commercial, and nonprofit insurance schemes, health maintenance organizations, and other agents managing prepaid medical and paramedical benefits (including the operating costs of these schemes).
  —Firms' expenditures on health, including both public and private enterprises, for medical care and health-enhancing benefits other than payment to social security.
  —Expenditures on health by nonprofit institutions serving mainly households.
  —Household out-of-pocket spending, including gratuities and in-kind payments made to health practitioners and suppliers of pharmaceuticals, therapeutic appliances, and other goods and services.

---

[26] OECD Health Data 2004, 1st edition: Note on General Comparability of Health Expenditure and Finance Data in OECD, http://www.irdes.fr/ecosante/OCDE/411.html.

NHA are essentially a standard set of tables that organize and present health expenditure information in a simple format (Partners for Health Reform*plus*, 2003a). Production of NHA requires extensive data collection from various ministries, donors, households, providers, and industry groups (e.g., private insurers, employers, pharmaceutical companies). Data come from a wide variety of sources, including government records (e.g., budget reports, tax reports, import and export statistics); other public records (e.g., ministry of health annual reports, financing and regulatory agency reports, NGO reports, academic studies, international agency reports); insurer records; provider records; and household surveys (World Health Organization, 2003). Information is obtained from multiple sources to triangulate (i.e., verify) data.

NHA are country data collection efforts supported by organizations such as WHO, PAHO, and PHR*plus*, which act as facilitators for country efforts and provide technical assistance and sometimes funding. WHO, PAHO, and PHR*plus* work collaboratively and have done so in many of the almost 70 countries that have conducted NHA. In addition, WHO, PAHO, and OECD assemble, organize, and cross-check country data and make them accessible to the wider public.

The work of OECD, WHO, PAHO, and PHR*plus* on NHA is discussed in more detail below. National HIV/AIDS Accounts and the use of NHA methodology for disease-specific expenditure analyses are also discussed.

OECD Health Data

Description

The Health Policy Unit of the OECD Directorate for Employment, Labour and Social Affairs (DELSA) collects data on health status and health care systems in the 30 OECD member countries.[27] DELSA examines employment and earning patterns, and its work on health focuses on ensuring an efficient and equitable delivery of high-quality health care services.[28] Work in the Health Policy Unit includes health policy analysis and health data collection, as well as studies on health and aging and international comparisons to assess the benefits and costs of pharmaceuticals. The Health Policy Unit also develops guidelines for improving international reporting of health expenditures through work on health accounting. The aim of its health policy work is to carry out cross-national studies of the performance of OECD health systems and to facilitate exchanges between member countries about their financing, delivery, and management of health services.[29]

OECD's *A System of Health Accounts* (SHA) manual contains guidelines for reporting health expenditures according to an international standard. It proposes a common boundary for health care, as well as a comprehensive and detailed structure for classifying the components of total expenditure on health (Organisation for Economic Co-operation and Development, 2000). It establishes a conceptual basis of statistical reporting rules and proposes a

---

[27] The OECD member countries are Australia, Austria, Belgium, Canada, Czech Republic, Denmark, Finland, France, Germany, Greece, Hungary, Iceland, Ireland, Italy, Japan, Korea, Luxembourg, Mexico, Netherlands, New Zealand, Norway, Poland, Portugal, Slovak Republic, Spain, Sweden, Switzerland, Turkey, United Kingdom, and United States.

[28] More information on OECD DELSA is available at http://www.oecd.org/about/0,2337,en_2649_33729_1_1_1_1_1,00.html.

[29] More information on OECD's Health Policy Unit is available at http://www.oecd.org/about/0,2337,en_2649_33929_1_1_1_1_1,00.html.

newly developed International Classification for Health Accounts (ICHA), which covers three dimensions: health care by function of care, providers of health care services, and sources of funding (Organisation for Economic Co-operation and Development, 2000). OECD member countries are currently at different stages in implementing the SHA.

The OECD Health Policy Unit has been publishing health statistics since the mid-1980s. OECD Health Data 2004 is the 13th edition of its electronic database on health systems.[30] This database, which contains data on several key aspects of the health care systems in the 30 OECD member countries, is a tool that can be used by health researchers and policy advisors in governments, the private sector, and the academic community to carry out comparative analyses and draw lessons from international comparisons of diverse health care systems.[31]

Data Collection

OECD Health Data is an interactive database covering over 1,200 indicators, for many of which the series goes back as far as 1960. Key items span the period from 1970 to 2001 or 2002, with selected Secretariat estimates for 2003. Data are presented in a demographic, economic, and social context.

The OECD health data are classified into ten main indicators (Organisation for Economic Co-operation and Development, 2004): (1) health status, (2) health care resources, (3) health care utilization, (4) expenditure on health, (5) health care financing, (6) social protection; (7) pharmaceutical market, (8) nonmedical determinants of health, (9) demographic references, and (10) economic references.

The two main indicators that deal with health expenditures—expenditure on health, and health care financing—are further broken down as follows:

1. Expenditure on health
   - National expenditure on health:
     — Total expenditure on health
     — Expenditure on personal health care
     — Expenditure on collective health care
     — Prevention and public health
     — Expenditure on health administration insurance
     — Expenditure on health-related functions
   - Expenditure on medical services
     — Total expenditure on medical services by functions
     — Expenditure on inpatient care
     — Expenditure on day care
     — Expenditure on outpatient care
     — Expenditure on home care
     — Expenditure on ancillary services

---

[30] OECD Health Data 2004 was developed jointly by the OECD Health Policy Unit and IRDES (Institut de Recherche et d'Etude en Economie de la Santé (formerly CREDES—Centre de Recherche, d'Etude et de Documentation en Economie de la Santé), a French research institute that specializes in health economics and health statistics.

[31] OECD, http://www.irdes.fr/ecosante/OCDE/31.html.

- Medical goods dispensed to outpatients
  — Total expenditure on medical goods
  — Pharmaceuticals & other medical non-durables
  — Therapeutic appliances & other medical durables
  — Current health expenditure by provider
- Expenditure by age and gender
- Price index
2. Health care financing
  - Health expenditure by sources of funds
    — General government, excluding social security
    — Social security schemes
    — Out-of-pocket payments (households)
    — Private insurance
    — Private insurance (other than social insurance)
    — Private social insurance
    — All other private funds (including rest of the world).

Not all OECD member countries report total expenditure on health according to the SHA methodology. Therefore, data reported in the OECD Health Data 2004 database are at varying levels of comparability (Organisation for Economic Co-operation and Development, 2004). The data for the database fall into four groups (Organisation for Economic Co-operation and Development, 2004):

1. Data from countries that report health expenditure information that closely follows the SHA methodology.
2. Data from countries that have "locally produced health accounts" that may or may not be comparable to the SHA definition of health care (e.g., Finland, New Zealand, Poland).
3. Data from countries that rely on national accounts for estimating health expenditure.[32]
4. Data consisting of estimates made by the OECD Secretariat based on the OECD National Account database. (Belgium is the only country in this group.)

Documentation of the definitions, national sources, and estimation methods used for each country is included in the database. Users of OECD Health Data 2004 can assess the quality of the data by consulting the sources and methods attached to each variable; the standard definition of the variable is provided, and any discrepancies between national data and the standard definitions are identified (Organisation for Economic Co-operation and Development, 2004). These definitions, sources, and discrepancies are subject to change in subsequent versions as they are refined over the years (Organisation for Economic Co-operation and Development, 2004).

There are important gaps with respect to international agreements on statistical methods that may affect cross-national comparisons of health care data (Organisation for Economic Co-operation and Development, 2004). The same term can refer to very different things among the 30 OECD countries, and efforts to develop homogeneity and standardized

---

[32] The countries that rely on national accounts to estimate health expenditure are Austria, Czech Republic, Greece, Iceland, Ireland, Italy, Luxembourg, Norway, Portugal, Slovak Republic, and Sweden.

health statistics are ongoing. The statistics contained in OECD Health Data 2004 reflect the situation at the time of release (Organisation for Economic Co-operation and Development, 2004). The comparability, consistency, and comprehensiveness of the data series have been improved with each successive release of the database (Organisation for Economic Co-operation and Development, 2004).

World Health Organization (WHO) National Health Accounts

Description

The World Health Organization (WHO) is the United Nations specialized agency for health. WHO's goal is to promote the best possible health for all people of the world. Health is defined in WHO's constitution as a state of complete physical, mental, and social well-being and not merely the absence of disease or infirmity.[33]

Since the early 1960s, WHO has supported the collection and analyses of health expenditure data.[34] Over the past five years, WHO has developed a systematic effort to measure resource flows in the health systems. The main products and outcomes to date are as follows:

- *World Health Report.* This WHO publication, put out annually since 1995, has contained selected measured ratios and levels of expenditures on health in all countries that are members of WHO since 2000. The report includes NHA indicators on total expenditure on health, broken into public and private expenditures. Selected components of public (social security expenditures on health) and private (health insurance and prepaid schemes and out-of-pocket expenditures) expenditures are presented. Data on external resources (i.e., expenditures on health originating outside the country, treated as a financing source) are also presented. The current report, *World Health Report 2004*, shows estimates for five years.[35]

- *WHO NHA Website.* In 2004, WHO launched an NHA Website that offers technical information and support to countries conducting NHA, as well as country-specific estimates on expenditures on health.[36] The Website provides information on resources available for conducting NHA studies in countries and offers technical support in the form of answers to questions from countries that are in the process of implementing NHA. The Website also provides the ratios available in the *World Health Report* and gives information on absolute values and sources of information on macro variables such as gross domestic product (GPD), general government expenditure, and average official and international dollar exchange rates. It also presents the various sources of information, along with the methods used to get those estimates.

- *NHA database (work in progress).* Published data are collated from several national and international sources and reports. Data are consolidated, triangulated, and harmonized in the NHA framework using international standard classifications and in

---

[33] WHO, http://www.who.int/about/en/.

[34] With the support of WHO, Able-Smith conducted the first major national studies of health expenditures in developing countries. For more information on these original studies, see Abel-Smith, 1963 and 1967.

[35] WHO's current and past editions of *World Health Report* are available at: http://www.who.int/whr/en/.

[36] The NHA Website is at http://www.who.int/nha/en.

agreement with national accounts standard procedures. Data are presented annually to each member state's ministry of health as part of a validation process. This process has proved useful in promoting national collation of data in a more standardized and systematic way and also helps in building national capacity. As part of the effort to reach better estimates, communication and collaboration with ministries and experts in the countries, national and international experts, and networks have increased extensively (through regional and country offices). While the information published is only for a few indicators, information is gathered wherever available to cover the whole set of NHA dimensions, including resource costs, financing sources, providers of care, health functions, pharmaceuticals, etc.

- *NHA framework (an incremental and consensual approach)*. To ensure a systematic, comprehensive, cost-effective, and comparable measurement of expenditure on health, the NHA framework has been discussed and improved. The framework is in line with the accounting principles of the *System of National Accounts 1993* of the UN and the OECD SHA. The resource flows cover the origins of funds (financing sources), the managers of funds and purchasers of health services (financing agents), the providers (producers of health services), the factors of production consumed in the process, the health services generated (functions), and the beneficiaries of the flow (by geopolitical entity, demographic, socioeconomic, and epidemiological status). The revised methods were reported in the *Guide to Producing National Health Accounts* (World Health Organization, World Bank, and United States Agency for International Development, 2003). Producing the guide entailed a three-year process with a steering and a technical committee that included institutional representatives and leading experts on NHA.
- *Capacity building.* WHO headquarters, along with WHO's six regional offices and 144 country and liaisons offices, and a network of partner organizations provide technical support to countries through training workshops and direct technical assistance to generate health expenditure information in agreement with the NHA framework. WHO supports the recurrent collection of updated expenditure data as part of an institutionalization process. The *Guide to Producing National Health Accounts* (World Health Organization, World Bank, and United States Agency for International Development, 2003), which is available in English, Arabic, and Russian, also contributes to capacity building and assists countries in measuring their national health expenditures.

Data Collection

WHO reports data on all financing agents along with external resources in its *World Health Report* and Website for 192 member states.[37] The indicators presented in the report and on the Website include (World Health Organization, 2004b):

- Total expenditure on health as a percentage of gross domestic product
- General government expenditure on health as a percentage of total expenditure on health
- Private sector expenditure on health as a percentage of total expenditure on health

---

[37] WHO, http://www.who.int/whr/2004/annex/country/en/.

- General government expenditure on health as a percentage of general government expenditure
- Social security funds as a percentage of general government expenditure on health
- Prepaid and risk-pooling plans as a percentage of private sector expenditure on health
- Private households' out-of-pocket payment as a percentage of private sector expenditure on health
- External resources on health as a percentage of total expenditure on health
- Total expenditure on health per capita at exchange rate
- Total expenditure on health per capita at international dollar rate
- General government expenditure on health per capita at exchange rate
- General government expenditure on health per capita at international dollar rate
- Gross domestic product (million national currency units [NCU])
- Exchange rate (NCU per US$)
- International dollar rate (NCU per international $)
- Total population (in thousands).

Though the data are reported only for the 16 indicators shown above, WHO collects information on more than 50 indicators on a regular basis, and collects information on more than 1,000 indicators wherever the information is available for the country. Additional, though not yet publishable, data have been collated for various other dimensions of resource flows, such as pharmaceutical expenditure, expenditure on hospitals, and inpatient care.

Data used to produce NHA estimates come from a wide variety of sources. In many countries, a great deal of information can be found in existing reports and national statistical projects (World Health Organization, 2004b). Sources of data include NHA reports, government records, other public records, insurer records, provider records, and household surveys. International reports are used to triangulate data obtained in national reports.

OECD and WHO work very closely together within a formal collaboration and agreement between the two institutions. OECD data are used for the OECD countries in the WHO NHA data reported in the annex of the *World Health Report* annually. WHO data are collated and analyzed in full collaboration between WHO headquarters and the six WHO regional offices. In addition, WHO health expenditure data for the past two years have been provided to World Bank for use in its *World Development Indicators* (WDI) report (see section below on this report for more detail on this health resource data collection).

Besides collating data and pursuing communication and discussion with country experts and responsible personnel, WHO makes data validation adjustments to correct biases, errors, and discontinuities in the data sources. Conceptual adjustments are made to bring figures in line with the NHA framework and definitions. Adjustments are made along with member states to ensure that estimates exhaustively cover the relevant entities in the health system of each country. National experts and institutional personnel are consulted to ensure that any adjustments made by WHO are in line with international rules and classifications.

The WHO NHA database is a work in progress. Estimates for already available indicators need to be improved and information for more NHA indicators must be collected. Work on measuring the reliability of estimates is in progress. Countrywide methodological information is being built up to be available in the future.

Approximately 70 countries have conducted NHA to date, and many other countries are beginning this type of activity. However, many countries have conducted only one study and no follow-up studies, which means trends cannot be monitored and analyzed. The ideal system would be one in which the flow of data is continuous—not one in which an NHA study is performed only once for special interest groups (largely donors). The great challenge is to ensure that the collection, compilation, and reporting of health expenditures is done on a routine basis and is sustainable.

Pan American Health Organization (PAHO) Health Accounts/National Health Accounts

Description

The Pan American Health Organization (PAHO), established in 1902, is an international public health agency that works to improve the health and living standards of the people of the Americas. PAHO is both the Regional Office for the Americas of WHO and the health organization of the Inter-American System. The member states of PAHO are all 35 countries in the Americas; Puerto Rico is an associate member. France, Netherlands, and the United Kingdom are participating states; Portugal and Spain are observer states.[38]

The health accounts (HA) and NHA compiled by PAHO are estimates of total national spending on health, health care services, and national health care systems. PAHO provides technical assistance to countries and maintains regional databases on national health care expenditures and on international trade in health-related goods and services (detailed in sections that follow).

As of June 2003, most Latin American and Caribbean (LAC) countries had carried out HA/NHA estimation at least once (estimation of national health care expenditures and sources of financing), up from 15 countries in 1999. Currently, most countries in the region have conducted at least an annual estimate of HA/NHA, several countries having HA/NHA for more than five years or periods. However, eight countries in the region still have not undertaken comprehensive HA/NHA estimations, and most of these are in the Caribbean.

The approaches and methodologies used to conduct HA/NHA estimations within the LAC region vary widely. So do the types of institutions involved in HA/NHA estimation, although ministries of health, statistical bureaus, and central banks form the majority.

PAHO began including a section on resources in health in its flagship publication, *Health in the Americas*, in 1994.[39] The 2002 edition of this publication, the most recent in the series, contains information covering 1997 through 2000 (Pan American Health Organization, 2002).

Data Collection

Several different types of data are collected for HA/NHA preparation: budget information about public sector spending, by institution, type of service, and input (such as personnel, medicine); information on private, out-of-pocket spending, which usually comes from analyses of household survey data; and data on other types of private spending, including expenditures by employers for insurance contributions and direct delivery of health services to workers. Specific sources of data vary from country to country.

---

[38] PAHO, http://www.paho.org/english/paho/What-PAHO.htm.

[39] *Health in the Americas* is published every four years.

Country studies on national health care expenditure and financing issues may be based on country-specific concepts, definitions, and accounting procedures, which are more relevant for national policy debate (administrative based studies), or on existing international standard concepts, classifications, and accounting procedures developed within the framework of the Government Finance Statistics Manual (IMF) and the UN SNA, which are more relevant for addressing public finance and international comparison issues related to national health systems expenditure and financing patterns (SNA-based studies; Pan American Health Organization, 2003).

PAHO also provides technical support and guidance in the development of pilot studies based on new and innovative HA/NHA approaches developed and promoted by other international organizations and by bilateral and multilateral agencies. These new approaches include

- OECD's System of Health Accounts (OECD's SHA)
- Harvard/PHR National Accounts approach (Harvard NHA)
- *Guide to Producing National Health Accounts* produced by WHO, World Bank, and USAID (released in June 2003).

The information presented for HA/NHA in PAHO's *Health in the Americas* series is for all health combined. More disaggregated data are needed, but they cannot be prepared without more resources. In addition, there are no systematic data on NGOs and nonprofit institutions serving households (NPISH), and it is difficult to obtain data on private health insurance.

Partners for Health Reform*plus* (PHR*plus*) National Health Accounts

Description

The Partners for Health Reform*plus* (PHR*plus*) project is the flagship project for the USAID Population, Health, and Nutrition (PHN) Center for health policy and systems strengthening in developing countries and countries in transition. PHR*plus* provides technical assistance to USAID in health care reform, health policy, management, health financing, and systems strengthening. PHR*plus* focuses on health policy, financing, organization, community participation, infectious disease surveillance, and information systems that support the management and delivery of appropriate health services. In addition, PHR*plus* conducts health systems research, implements performance monitoring and results tracking, provides training and capacity development, and is responsible for strategic documentation and transfer of experiences in health policy and systems strengthening.

PHR*plus* is funded for the five-year period of 2000 to 2005. It builds on two previous projects led by Abt Associates for USAID: the Health Financing and Sustainability project (1989–1995) and the Partnerships for Health Reform (PHR) project (1995–2000). PHR*plus* is implemented by Abt Associates, Inc., in collaboration with Development Associates, Inc.; Emory University Rollins School of Public Health; Philoxenia International Travel, Inc.; Program for Appropriate Technology in Health; Social Sectors Development Strategies, Inc.; Training Resources Group; Tulane University School of Public Health and Tropical Medicine; and University Research Co., LLC.

PHR*plus* works in over 25 countries spanning four regions of the world. It has close working relationships with NGOs and USAID cooperating agencies and with international and developing country partner organizations, including World Bank, WHO, UNICEF, bilateral donors, Private Voluntary Organizations (PVOs), foundations, universities, and host country government agencies.

PHR*plus* has provided support and technical assistance to countries conducting NHA for the past eight years. It focuses on capacity building and institutionalization of NHA in developing countries and on a variety of innovative NHA-based analyses. PHR*plus* has worked very closely with several donors on the development and institutionalization of NHA, including WHO, SIDA, World Bank, and EU. PHR, PHR*plus*, and other donors have supported national governments in more than 51 low- and middle-income countries in conducting, analyzing, and considering the implications of NHA.[40]

Data Collection

NHA conducted with the support of PHR*plus* track detailed information on health resource flows from the source of funding (e.g., government, donors, households), to the distribution to financing agents (e.g., ministry of health, ministry of education, social security, out-of-pocket), and all the way down to the level of functions (e.g., inpatient care, drugs). NHA rely on information from several sources, including: (1) secondary sources that already exist, such as studies from the ministry of health, ministry of finance, and universities; (2) government budget documents; (3) surveys/questionnaires to collect information not readily available from other sources; (4) annual donor reports; (5) household surveys. Information is obtained from multiple sources to allow cross-checking (triangulation) of findings.

Many times it is necessary to rely on estimates of expenditures because the government reports on spending are not detailed enough. Some countries have a decentralized government, so it is necessary to include information obtained at the local level to get accurate expenditure flows.

Data on out-of-pocket expenditures by households are not always available. It can also be difficult to obtain information from the private sector (i.e., industry, insurance, NGOs) since they are not required to make their spending information public.

Regional AIDS Initiative for Latin America and the Caribbean (SIDALAC) National HIV/AIDS Accounts

Description

SIDALAC is implemented by the Mexican Health Foundation. In 1995, World Bank asked the Mexican Health Foundation to execute this program. In 1996, UNAIDS came on board as a co-sponsor with World Bank. SIDALAC is now part of UNAIDS and is funded primarily by World Bank and UNAIDS.[41]

SIDALAC is a regional initiative focused on economics and HIV/AIDS. It has the following general objectives:

---

[40] PHR*plus*, http://www.phrplus.org/focus_new8.html.

[41] The majority of National HIV/AIDS Accounts conducted in Latin America from 1999 through 2002 were funded by the European Commission.

- To develop research projects that provide useful information for strategic planning in the prevention of HIV/AIDS and other sexually transmitted diseases (STDs) and the provision of adequate health care for affected individuals.
- To widely disseminate the results of such research projects and to promote the interchange of country experiences and lessons learned.[42]

Data Collection

One of the main activities conducted by SIDALAC is the estimation of national AIDS expenditures (National HIV/AIDS Accounts) in 20 countries in Latin America and the Caribbean, and in Ghana and Burkina Faso.[43] *National HIV/AIDS Accounts* is the term applied to the "systematic, periodical and exhaustive accounting of the expenditures and financing from the public and private sectors that are directed to the prevention and treatment of people with HIV/AIDS" (Regional AIDS Initiative for Latin America and the Caribbean, 2001, p. 12). The main purpose of the National HIV/AIDS Accounts is to influence policy formulation and decisionmaking and to improve the allocation of resources for HIV/AIDS.

SIDALAC National HIV/AIDS Accounts track both health and nonhealth (e.g., research, training, policy dialogue, advocacy, and mitigation of HIV/AIDS—orphans, nutritional supplements, etc.) expenditures. Nonhealth expenditures are a small percentage of the total, since the cost of care, anti-retrovirals, and prevention strategies (e.g., blood banks, condoms) is very high in comparison. SIDALAC also tracks private, public, and international expenditures. Private expenditures include industry/private corporations, insurance, NGOs (domestic and international), and out-of-pocket spending; public expenditures include ministries of health and social security; and international expenditures include both multilateral and bilateral donors.

The main questions addressed by National HIV/AIDS Accounts are (Regional AIDS Initiative for Latin America and the Caribbean, 2001):

- In what proportion do government, social security funds, the nonprofit sector, households, businesses, and international cooperation agencies contribute to HIV/AIDS activities?
- What kinds of service providers are receiving resources earmarked for HIV/AIDS prevention, treatment, and administration?
- What programs and services receive funds and in what proportions?
- How is the funding distributed among geographic zones and human groups?

SIDALAC is interested in capacity building. It gives people hands-on training so they can set up continuous information systems on resource tracking. Once the system is set up, some countries will continue to track HIV/AIDS expenditures on their own and some will need more funding.

---

[42] SIDALAC, http://www.sidalac.org.mx/english/whatis.htm.

[43] The 20 countries in Latin America and the Caribbean in which SIDALAC has established National HIV/AIDS Accounts are Argentina, Belize, Bolivia, Brazil, Chile, Colombia, Costa Rica, Cuba, Dominican Republic, El Salvador, Guatemala, Guyana, Honduras, Mexico, Nicaragua, Panama, Paraguay, Peru, Uruguay, and Venezuela.

SIDALAC is trying to standardize the collection and presentation of data. The presentation is similar to the OECD SHA and WHO NHA, but with different identification of functions and services for HIV/AIDS.

SIDALAC is tracking both monies and services, with services translated into or measured in money (the cost of the service being estimated if there are no records of money spent). Data are collected by a combination of interviews, surveys, and primary sources. (Household surveys are not often used, because they are too expensive.) SIDALAC depends on the information already available in a country.

While most of the information SIDALAC collects is very detailed, different levels of detail are presented in the various reports that SIDALAC prepares. For example, the overall report on all countries is less detailed than are the reports about individual countries. National AIDS Program authorities have the most-detailed figures.

The data collected by SIDALAC provide a retrospective review of the two previous years (e.g., in 1998 SIDALAC launched an initiative to look at 1997 and 1998). The most recent year for which SIDALAC has data is 2002 (and this is only for 11 of the 20 countries for which it has estimates). It is moving to a more continuous system, so that the first quarter of the year will have information from the previous year.

SIDALAC has collected good information on most Latin American countries. It has a sequence of two to four years of resource tracking data for most countries, and six to seven years for some. Data are not as good for Caribbean countries—there are more difficulties in capacity building. In March 2004, SIDALAC, in collaboration with PHR*plus*, began programs in Africa and Eastern Europe.

It is difficult to obtain information about spending at the local level of government, especially in countries such as Brazil, Argentina, and Mexico. Many African countries also have expenditures at the district level, and these, too, are hard to track. Obtaining information about out-of-pocket expenditures and about expenditures for nontraditional providers of service (e.g., healers) is also difficult.

It is also difficult to measure additionality. Much of the data are totaled and reported at an aggregated level, so details about what the money was spent on are lacking.

Partners for Health Reform*plus* (PHR*plus*) HIV/AIDS, Malaria, and Reproductive Health Subanalyses

PHR*plus* has helped countries use the NHA framework to track resource flows for HIV/AIDS in Rwanda, Kenya, and Zambia, and is helping several other countries use this approach. In addition, the NHA methodology is being used to capture expenditures in other disease categories, such as malaria, and in reproductive health. Furthermore, WHO, along with other partners, including PHR*plus*, has initiated a process to standardize disease-specific subanalyses.

PHR*plus* is collaborating with SIDALAC on the tracking of HIV/AIDS expenditures, and the two organizations are mapping their methodologies onto each other. Though SIDALAC and PHR*plus* started from different perspectives in developing a methodology for tracking HIV/AIDS expenditures using the OECD SHA framework, they have arrived at remarkably similar methodologies. PHR*plus* is also collaborating on HIV/AIDS subanalyses with a number of other organizations, such as USAID, WHO, and UNAIDS.

World Health Organization (WHO) Disease-Specific Expenditures

WHO is in the process of producing a supplement to the *Guide to Producing National Health Accounts* that outlines the necessary framework for tracking resources for diseases and other health expenditure priorities. Special efforts are in progress to measure disease-specific expenditures as well as additionality for HIV/AIDS, tuberculosis, and malaria. WHO has also funded country case studies to address the question of additionality and the possibility of using NHA studies to monitor these indicators.

Data on Donor Aid and Country-Level Expenditures/Activities: Other

World Development Indicators (WDI) Database

Description

World Development Indicators (WDI) is World Bank's premier annual statistical report about development. WDI 2004 includes approximately 800 indicators in 87 tables, organized in six sections: world view, people, environment, economy, states and markets, and global links. The tables cover 152 economies and 14 country groups, with basic indicators for a further 55 economies. The print edition of WDI provides a current overview of data from the previous few years. Time-series data from 1960 onward are available on the WDI CD-ROM version or WDI Online.[44]

Data Collection

WDI Online, available via paid subscription, provides direct access to 575 development indicators, with time series for 208 countries and 18 country groups from 1960 to 2003, where data are available (2003 data are available for selected indicators only). World Bank provides free access to WDI Online through Data Query, which offers a segment of the WDI database.[45] Data Query contains five years of data (1998 to 2002) for 54 indicators for 208 countries and 18 groups.

The 575 indicators are broken down into the following categories: people, environment, economy, states and markets, and global links. The people category has a subgroup of indicators on health:

- Births attended by health staff (percentage of total)
- Health expenditure per capita (current US$)
- Health expenditure, private (percentage of GDP)
- Health expenditure, public (percentage of GDP)
- Health expenditure, total (percentage of GDP)
- Hospital beds (per 1,000 people)
- Immunization, DPT (diphtheria, pertussis, and tetanus) (percentage of children under 12 months)
- Immunization, measles (percentage of children under 12 months)
- Improved water source (percentage of population with access)

---

[44] http://www.worldbank.org/data/wdi2004/index.htm.

[45] Available at http://devdata.worldbank.org/data-query/.

- Physicians (per 1,000 people)
- Improved sanitation facilities (percentage of population with access).

World Bank is not a primary data collection agency for most issues other than living standards surveys and debt. The primary data collectors are usually national statistical agencies, central banks, and customs services.[46] Differences in the methods and conventions used by the primary data collectors may give rise to significant discrepancies over time both among and within countries (World Bank, 2004). Delays in reporting data and the use of old surveys as the base for current estimates may severely compromise the quality of national data (World Bank, 2004).

Data quality is improving in some countries; however, many developing countries lack the resources to train and maintain the skilled staff and to obtain the equipment needed to measure and report demographic, economic, and environmental trends in an accurate and timely way (World Bank, 2004). World Bank is working with bilateral and other multilateral agencies to fund and participate in technical assistance projects to improve statistical organization and basic data methods, collection, and dissemination (World Bank, 2004).

National Health Care Expenditure Database (NHExp Database)

Description

The National Health Care Expenditure (NHExp) Database was developed and is maintained by PAHO to collect regional data on comparable international indicators of national health care expenditures.[47] Information is presented in two ways: as graphs and tables providing snapshots of the data by different categories and groups of countries, and as a database with estimates from 1980 through 1998 for the Americas.

Data Collection

The NHExp Database contains estimates from 48 Latin American and Caribbean (LAC) countries and territories on public and private expenditures in health, including

- Public expenditures—expenditures by governments, including social insurance funds and other public sector institutions.
- Private expenditures—out-of-pocket expenditures by households in health related goods and services (direct) and in health insurance and pre-paid health plans (indirect), and expenditures on health by NPISH. There are no estimates on health expenditures by financial and nonfinancial corporations.

The NHExp Database also contains time series of macroeconomic variables (e.g., GDP, population, exchange rates, and estimates on total government expenditures) commonly used for deriving national health expenditure indicators and projections: per capita expenditures, share of health expenditures as a percentage of GDP or gross national income (GNI), income-expenditure elasticity, and conversion to purchasing power parity (PPP). The

---

[46] For the last two years, World Bank has largely used WHO NHA figures in its world development indicators.

[47] PAHO, http://newweb.www.paho.org/English/DPM/SHD/HP/nhexp-datab-intr.htm.

estimates of national health care expenditures in the NHExp Database are based on the guidelines of the UN's SNA, the IMF's Government Finance Statistics Manual, and new international standards developed within the framework of the UN Statistical Commission, as well as on the Statistical Conference of the Americas (SCAECLAC).[48]

The definition of *public health expenditure* is problematic, given the variability of the health systems and national budgeting structures of each LAC country or territory in the database. For most countries in the region, data on central government health expenditures exist in some form or other. These figures are often produced by national financial authorities and ministries of health for international agencies such as IMF, World Bank, IDB, and the UN, as well as for their own analysis. Expenditures at other levels of government (state, provincial, municipal, etc.) are less well documented but are becoming increasingly important in the region. In addition, the quality and availability of data on social security health expenditures vary significantly from country to country, and these data are often years out of date.

Finally, private expenditures on health are relatively undocumented, with no data available for a large percentage of countries in the region. These expenditures encompass not only household payments—both direct payments for health care received and indirect payments through health insurance—but also corporate health expenditures, as well as the health expenditures of community, religious, and charitable organizations and of other NGOs.

Data Base of Trade in Health Related Goods and Services in the Americas

Description

PAHO's *Data Base of Trade in Health Related Goods and Services in the Americas* is a report that contains information on statistics of international trade in health related commodities in countries of the American region (Pan American Health Organization and World Health Organization, 2003). It presents information on the estimated value of total exports and imports of health related goods or commodities for Canada, United States, and countries of the Latin American and Caribbean region for 1994 through 2000. It also specifically tracks the value of the exports and imports of two broad components of the international trade in health related products: pharmaceutical, medicinal chemical and botanical products, and medical and surgical equipment and orthopedic appliances, as classified in the International Standard Industrial Classification (ISIC), Revision 3 (ISIC Rev. 3).[49] All the statistical information is presented in current U.S. dollars.

Data Collection

The main source of data for the *Data Base of Trade in Health Related Goods and Services in the Americas* is DATAINTAL 3.1 (2002)—Trade Statistics System for the Western Hemisphere.[50] DATAINTAL is a system of import and export statistics of countries in the Americas. It was designed to meet the needs of decisionmakers, researchers, and analysts concerned with international trade, and is a tool for analyzing historical data, looking at trends, gauging

---

[48] PAHO, http://newweb.www.paho.org/English/DPM/SHD/HP/nhexp-datab-intr.htm.

[49] PAHO, http://www.paho.org/English/DPM/SHD/HP/trade-datab.htm.

[50] DATAINTAL is available at http://www.iadb.org/intal/ingles/bdi/i-dataintalweb.htm.

the competition, or discovering potential new markets. It consists of programs and databases that allow users to query the data and obtain current and historical trade data in a table format that can be printed or imported into other programs. DATAINTAL was developed by the Institute for the Integration of Latin America and the Caribbean (INTAL), in Buenos Aires, Argentina, and the Unit of Statistics and Quantitative Analysis, both of which are units of the IDB's Department of Integration and Regional Programs.

INTAL collects trade data from official government organizations that produce national trade statistics and from international organizations. INTAL began collecting trade data in 1984, mainly for internal use by the IDB. In 1990, INTAL began distributing the data to foreign trade research and promotion organizations in several Latin American countries; in 1998, the first DATAINTAL version in CD-ROM format was widely distributed.

The information in PAHO's *Data Base of Trade in Health Related Goods and Services in the Americas* covers only 1994 to 2000. The only year for which there is information for all 29 countries in the DATAINTAL database is 1997, so 1997 was used as the reference year.[51] The information or averages shown for 1994 do not include figures from Bahamas and Panama, which account for 1.1 percent of the total trade exchange (exports plus imports) in health goods in 1997. Similarly, statistics of 2000 do not include figures from Bahamas, Barbados, Belize, Dominica, Grenada, Jamaica, Panama, Saint Kitts, Saint Lucia, Saint Vincent, and Trinidad. The participation of these countries in the total trade exchange of 1997 is around 2.3 percent.

Institute for Democracy in South Africa (Idasa) Budget Information Service (BIS) Budget Briefs and Reports

Description

The Institute for Democracy in South Africa (Idasa) Budget Information Service (BIS) uses data and budget information published by the South African government to analyze revenue and expenditure impacts on the lives of low-income, poor, and vulnerable communities. BIS performs issue-based and sector analyses of public spending on HIV/AIDS, health, education, social welfare, human resource and infrastructure development, and local government finance, as well as research on policy and budget allocations affecting vulnerable groups, such as children and women. The BIS units publish their budget analyses in several types of publications, including budget briefs, occasional papers, and books. This independent research is used to enhance the role of civil society organizations in their pro-poor and rights-based advocacy work, to inform parliamentarians in their oversight and monitoring of government departments, to engage government officials, and to influence and advocate budget decisions.[52]

BIS is composed of several units/projects that track public spending on health care and are involved in training and advocacy, including

- Children's Budget Unit

---

[51] The 29 countries are Argentina, Bahamas, Barbados, Belize, Bolivia, Brazil, Canada, Chile, Colombia, Costa Rica, Dominica, Ecuador, El Salvador, Grenada, Guatemala, Honduras, Jamaica, Mexico, Nicaragua, Panama, Paraguay, Peru, Saint Kitts, Saint Lucia, Saint Vincent, Trinidad, Uruguay, United States, and Venezuela.

[52] Idasa, http://www.idasact.org.za/bis/.

- Sector Budget Analysis Unit
- AIDS Budget Unit.

Data Collection

The BIS Children's Budget Unit was established in 1995 with the objective of conducting research and disseminating information on the South African government's budgeting for children in South Africa. It analyzes resource allocation by government for children in South Africa with respect to policy and legislation for children and government expenditure and service delivery for child poverty alleviation. The Children's Budget Unit has published several books focused on government spending on children in five key sectors: health, education, welfare, policing, and justice.

The BIS Sector Budget Analysis Unit (previously the Provincial Fiscal Analysis Unit) started off in 1995 by mapping the new South African intergovernmental system. This unit was concerned with analyzing government budget allocations and implementations that contribute to eradicating poverty and inequity in South Africa and Africa, and that foster human development to enlarge people's choices and raise levels of well-being.[53] In subsequent years, the Sector Budget Analysis Unit built on this basic work by deepening its sector specific research capacity in health, education, and welfare, with a particular focus on provincial spending where the majority of social sector service delivery takes place.

The Sector Budget Analysis Unit recently broadened its scope to include national and local government and a wider range of sectors (e.g., housing, land, economic sector). This will enable the unit to provide a more comprehensive overview of the impact of public spending on the lives and well-being of poor people and to respond more swiftly to requests for budget information and research in the health, education, and welfare sectors.

The BIS AIDS Budget Unit provides research and analysis on the public finance issues related to government's response to HIV/AIDS. It monitors targeted allocations for HIV/AIDS interventions in the national and provincial budgets and analyzes the indirect impact of the epidemic on the public sector budget. It conducts an annual HIV/AIDS budget analysis, which is a comprehensive list of national and provincial allocations for HIV/AIDS, and publishes budget briefs on relevant topics.[54]

In November 2003, the AIDS Budget Unit published a report, *Budgeting for HIV/AIDS in South Africa: Report on Intergovernmental Funding Flows for an Integrated Response in the Social Sector* (Hickey, Ndlovu, and Guthrie, 2003), that examines provincial capacity and spending procedures for HIV/AIDS programs and gives recommendations on the most-effective ways to channel funds to the provinces to fight the epidemic. A companion document, "Where is HIV/AIDS in the Budget? Survey of 2002 Provincial Social Sector Budgets" (Ndlovu, 2003), identifies (based on desk study and provincial interviews) HIV/AIDS specific allocations in provincial education, social development, and health department budgets.

In addition to regularly analyzing HIV/AIDS budgeting and expenditures in South Africa, the AIDS Budget Unit and FUNDAR Center for Analysis and Research jointly coordinated an international comparative analysis of HIV/AIDS expenditures and budgeting in

---

[53] Idasa, http://www.idasact.org.za/bis/.

[54] Idasa, http://www.idasact.org.za/bis/.

nine countries: Argentina, Chile, Ecuador, Mexico, Namibia, Nicaragua, Mozambique, Kenya, and South Africa. This study, undertaken by NGO research institutes in each country, compares how governments are funding the fight against HIV/AIDS and builds capacity for HIV/AIDS budget analysis in the participating countries. The results of the study were discussed by researchers during a one-day meeting held in Benoni, South Africa, on September 20, 2004, and were published in an Idasa report entitled *Funding the Fight: Budgeting for HIV/AIDS in Developing Countries* (Guthrie and Hickey, 2004).

Immunization Financing Database

Description

In July 2004, the Immunization Financing Database, a comprehensive database on immunization spending and financing developed by the Global Alliance for Vaccines and Immunization (GAVI) Financing Task Force (FTF), became available online with information from 22 countries.[55] The FTF, a team of technical experts from Abt Associates/PHR*plus*, the Children's Vaccine Program, UNICEF, PAHO, the Vaccine Fund, World Bank, and WHO, began working on the Immunization Financing Database in November 2001.

Data Collection

The Immunization Financing Database provides information about baselines and trends on immunization spending and financial flows. This information will help the FTF fulfill its responsibilities of increasing the understanding of why there is inadequate funding for vaccines and immunization in the poorest countries, and identifying strategies to improve the capacity of governments, donors, and development banks to finance these needs.

The information in the database is derived from the detailed data on past and future costing and financing that countries submit in their Financial Sustainability Plan (FSP) to GAVI at the midpoint in their funding from the Vaccine Fund.[56] All eligible countries are required to prepare an FSP and to provide regular updates through the annual progress reporting mechanism.[57] Data are made available in the database after the FSP has been reviewed and accepted by the GAVI independent review committee and the data have been reviewed and analyzed by the immunization financing database team.[58] Future updates of existing data in the database will be done through the GAVI Annual Progress Report (APR) mechanism and throughout the implementation phase of countries' FSPs.

The data reported in the FSPs include detailed information by cost category and by funding source. The cost category covers recurrent costs and capital costs. Recurrent costs are vaccines, injection supplies, personnel, transport, cold chain maintenance, building overheads, training, social mobilization, monitoring, surveillance, and information, education, and communication (IEC); capital costs are vehicles, cold chain equipment, and buildings.

---

[55] As of July 9, 2004, the Immunization Financing Database is available online at http://www.who.int/immunization_financing/data/en/.

[56] The Vaccine Fund is a financing mechanism designed to help the GAVI alliance achieve its objectives by raising new resources and swiftly channeling them to developing countries.

[57] GAVI eligible countries are governments in the 75 poorest countries with GNI below US$1000 (from http://www.pasteur.fr/actu/presse/press/02GAVI-E.htm).

[58] WHO Immunization Financing, http://www.who.int/immunization_financing/data/about/availability/en/.

Retrospective data on costing and financing are required for two years, including a year before GAVI and the Vaccine Fund (baseline year). Prospective data are required for two periods (about eight years): Period 1 includes all the remaining years with Vaccine Fund support, and period 2 comprises the immediate years following the end of Vaccine Fund support. A costing, financing, and gap analysis tool has been developed to help countries prepare this information for their FSP.

It is difficult for countries to determine the donor country for the bilateral aid they receive through SWAp programs and national budget support. Therefore, countries are asked to report in FSP only the source of financing closest to the end use. This means that funding from bilateral donors to multilateral agencies, to SWAp programs, and to national treasuries for budget support is not attributed to the donor countries.[59] In addition, the FSP focuses on program-specific costs, which means that the data do not account for the national government's contribution to such key inputs as personnel and facilities, which are shared across multiple health programs.[60]

Country Response Information System (CRIS)

Description

UNAIDS is the main advocate for global action on HIV/AIDS. The goal of UNAIDS is to lead, strengthen, and support an expanded response aimed at preventing the transmission of HIV, providing care and support, reducing the vulnerability of individuals and communities to HIV/AIDS, and alleviating the impact of the epidemic.[61]

In response to the need for improved information and analysis at national and global levels, UNAIDS has developed the Country Response Information System (CRIS) to facilitate the systematic collection, storage, analysis, retrieval, and dissemination of information on a country's response to HIV/AIDS (Joint United Nations Programme on HIV/AIDS, 2003). CRIS is designed to house information collected on indicators, resources, and scientific research relating to HIV/AIDS. CRIS, which will be operational in more than 100 countries by 2005, provides a structure for countries to collect information relative to the epidemic, the response, and the impact, including epidemiological information; strategic planning, costing, and coordination capacities; budget allocations to AIDS programming and other resource flows; and project implementation rates.[62] CRIS allows direct country-to-country exchange of information and facilitates better collection, storage, analysis, and dissemination of information.

In addition, UNAIDS contracts with NIDI, SIDALAC, and other data collection organizations to provide an overall analysis of resource flows for HIV/AIDS. In 2002, UNAIDS also established a Global Resource Tracking Consortium for AIDS, composed of international experts who track the financial expenditures on HIV/AIDS at national and international levels. Partners in the Global Resource Tracking Consortium for AIDS include ABT Associates Inc./PHR*plus*, International AIDS Vaccine Initiative, Alliance for Mircrobi-

---

[59] WHO Immunization Financing, http://www.who.int/immunization_financing/data/about/limitations/en/.

[60] WHO Immunization Financing, http://www.who.int/immunization_financing/data/about/limitations/en/.

[61] UNAIDS, http://www.unaids.org/EN/about+unaids/what+is+unaids.asp.

[62] UNAIDS, http://www.unaids.org/EN/in+focus/monitoringevaluation/country+response+information+system.asp.

cide Development, FCAA, Futures Group, GFATM, Kaiser Family Foundation, Idasa, Instituto Nacional de Salud Publica (INSP), OECD, Resource Flows for Population Activities and AIDS, SIDALAC, UNFPA, WHO, and UNAIDS.

Data Collection

CRIS includes a core of standardized information on the HIV/AIDS situation and the response in participating countries, facilitating analysis of that information. CRIS contains three databases: the Indicator Database (IND), the Project Resource Tracking (PRT) database, and the Research Inventory Database (RID).

The IND, the first component of CRIS to be operational, supports the collection and analysis of local indicators of the HIV/AIDS epidemic. It consists of core fields and free fields. The core fields have predetermined definitions installed with the database, which correspond to the indicators for measuring follow-up to the UNGASS on HIV/AIDS Declaration of Commitment.[63] The collection of a standardized core of indicators will allow for improved local analysis and provide a better picture of the status of the national response to the HIV/AIDS epidemic. The free fields will allow the system to be customized to meet local needs.

The PRT was developed to be complementary to the IND. It was released in August 2004, and training and support activities will be provided over the next year to maximize its use at the country level. The purpose of the PRT is to facilitate improved monitoring and evaluation of the national response to HIV/AIDS through the financial tracking of projects and programs. The PRT will allow the tracking of resources and activities being undertaken in-country and the analysis of funding and program gaps by any combination of parameters, including time frame, geographic area, target population, type of project, and organization.

The PRT was designed to be a flexible report and analysis tool. Information in the PRT can be assembled into reports using any combination of the following criteria (Joint United Nations Programme on HIV/AIDS, 2003):

1. Subnational functional level, i.e., province or district
2. Executing/implementing organization or type of that organization (government ministry, provincial ministry, UN agency, NGO, etc.)
3. Resource provider (donor)
4. Planned or actual start and/or end dates for projects
5. Project budget range
6. Whether the project is fully funded or underfunded
7. Whether projects have actually begun
8. Target populations' gender, age group, occupation, and/or ethnicity
9. A variety of activity descriptions or keywords that more fully describe projects
10. How a project fulfills the goals in the National Strategic Plan.

---

[63] UNAIDS, http://www.unaids.org/EN/in+focus/monitoringevaluation/country+response+information+system/indicator+database. asp.

The RID, which is currently being field tested in Bangladesh and Uganda, will enable countries to track research related to HIV/AIDS and STDs.[64] The goal of RID is to enhance the collaboration among decisionmakers and program planners, researchers, research institutions, and funding agencies in order to strengthen developing-country research capacity and enhance the role of research in informing responses to the epidemic. RID will facilitate the collection of global data on research funding agencies and research awards. This information can then be compared to the actual research conducted in countries.

The country-level CRIS will be complemented by a Global Response Information Database (GRID). Selected data from CRIS from all countries will be housed centrally in GRID by the UNAIDS Secretariat. Data from local CRIS systems will be aggregated and presented on the GRID Website. Countries will be encouraged to share the core fields of CRIS with the UNAIDS Secretariat so that all countries' core fields can be replicated on GRID. The GRID Website will provide tools to facilitate the creation of reports and pursue more-detailed analysis of global data from CRIS. GRID will also provide a referral point to national CRIS systems for further and more-detailed information about national epidemics, the responses being undertaken, and the impacts of these upon the respective country. GRID will be constructed so that when data are updated at the national level in CRIS, the changes will be reflected on the global site on a regular basis. GRID will allow for data searches across countries. It will also maximize links with other information systems of the UN system and other strategic partners.

Examples of Other Types of Databases

Several donors maintain databases that track their own activities. These databases usually contain specific information about the projects/programs funded by these donors. Some of these databases are online, searchable, and publicly available—e.g., World Bank Projects Database and GFATM Funded Programs Database—both of which are described briefly below.

In addition, there are several databases that contain specialized information:

- Databases tracking contraception:
  - UNFPA has maintained a database since 1990 that contains country-specific information reported by donors on the type, quantity, and total cost of contraceptives they provided to reproductive health programs in developing countries. Information in the database is the basis of an annual publication by UNFPA on donor support for reproductive health commodities.[65]
  - RH Interchange tracks procurement data on reproductive health commodities (condoms, contraceptives, and other essential reproductive health supplies) by country, method, and donor for the three major donors of reproductive health

---

[64] Funding for the development of the RID has been provided by the Office of AIDS Research at the National Institutes of Health (http://www.unaids.org/EN/in+focus/monitoringevaluation/country+response+information+system/research+inventory+database.asp).

[65] UNFPA's most recent report on reproductive health commodities, "Donor Support for Contraceptives and Condoms for STI/HIV Prevention 2001," is available at http://www.unfpa.org/upload/lib_pub_file/192_filename_contraceptives_01.pdf.

supplies: International Planned Parenthood Federation (IPPF), UNFPA, and USAID.[66]

- Databases/reports tracking pharmaceuticals and medical equipment:

—IMS Health, a private sector consulting firm is probably the best source of data on U.S. pharmaceutical production, sales, and flows from drug manufacturers, retail and institutional pharmacies, hospitals, wholesalers, prescribers, and others. IMS has data from over 90 countries covering all stages of a drug's life cycle and is willing to do special studies for a fee (starting at $2,000).

—Partnership for Quality Medical Donations (PQMD) is an alliance of private voluntary organizations and medical product manufacturers dedicated to raising standards of medical donations to underserved populations and disaster victims around the world. PQMD sponsored the first systematic assessment of U.S. pharmaceutical donations. Conducted by the Harvard School of Public Health, this study outlined policy recommendations to improve the donation process.

—UNICEF provides supplies for children within the organization's priority areas of immunization, fighting HIV/AIDS, early childhood development, education, and child protection in emergencies.[67] UNICEF's Supply Division is responsible for overseeing the organization's global procurement and logistics operation, including bulk purchasing and distribution of medicines and medical supplies. The Supply Division Annual Report 2003 details how supplies are used and shows UNICEF's key commodities, where supplies are bought, and where they are used.[68]

—WHO has an NHA database that contains aggregate information on pharmaceuticals, but this database is not publicly available. Information gathered for the NHA database covers the whole set of NHA dimensions (wherever available), including resource costs, financing sources, providers of care, health functions, and pharmaceuticals.

—United Nations Conference on Trade and Development (UNCTAD) focuses on the integrated treatment of trade and development and the interrelated issues of finance, technology, investment, and sustainable development.[69] The UNCTAD Handbook of Statistics On-line is a database that provides a comprehensive collection of statistical data relevant to the analysis of international trade, foreign direct investment, and development for individual countries and for regional and economic groupings.[70] It contains information on international merchandise trade, trade and commodity price indices, structure of international trade by region and by product, and international trade in services, including aggregate information on the imports and exports of medicinal and pharmaceutical products and medical instruments.

---

[66] RH Interchange, http://www.rhsupplies.org/textonly/rhinterchange/rhinterchange.html.

[67] UNICEF, http://www.unicef.org/supply/index.html.

[68] UNICEF's Supply Division Annual Report 2003 is available at http://www.unicef.org/supply/SupplyDivisionAnnualReport2003.pdf.

[69] UNCTAD, http://www.unctad.org/Templates/Page.asp?intItemID=1530&lang=1.

[70] UNCTAD, http://www.unctad.org/Templates/Page.asp?intItemID=1890&lang=1.

— DATAINTAL has databases (online and CD-ROM versions) that contain import and export statistics for countries in the Americas. It allows users to query the data and obtain current and historical trade data.

— ECRI is an independent nonprofit health services research agency with a wide range of specialized products and services, many of which are provided within the framework of membership programs focused on health care technology (e.g., planning, procurement, and management). ECRI's PriceGuide™ is a member-searchable database of discounted prices of record actually paid for a wide range of single-use medical products, plus a clinical equivalency testing service.[71]

World Bank Projects Database

The Projects Database provides access to basic information on all of World Bank lending projects from 1947, when World Bank started operations, to the present.[72] It was created to help make World Bank's lending more transparent to the public and its partners and to encourage broader participation in the projects that World Bank finances.

All World Bank projects are classified according to one to five sectors, which are a high-level grouping of economic activities based on the types of goods or services produced. The UN classification of economic sectors was used as a point of reference.

The Projects Database can be searched by country, region, sector, priority/goal, or theme. Searching by sectors or themes provides access to the health related projects funded by World Bank. The human development sector comprises the following themes:

- Child health
- Other communicable diseases
- Injuries and noncommunicable diseases
- Nutrition and food security
- Population and reproductive health
- HIV/AIDS
- Health system performance.

The Global Fund Funded Programs Database

The main purpose of the GFATM is to attract, manage, and disburse resources to fight AIDS, tuberculosis, and malaria. Since 2001, GFATM has attracted US$4.7 billion in pledges and contributions; pledges have been made through 2008. In its first two rounds of grantmaking, it has committed US$1.5 billion in funding to support 154 programs in 93 countries worldwide.[73]

The Funded Programs Database contains information about grant commitments and disbursements of GFATM grants:[74]

---

[71] ECRI (formerly the Emergency Care Research Institute), http://www.ecri.org/Products_and_Services/Membership_Programs/Membership_Programs.aspx.

[72] The Projects Database is available at http://web.worldbank.org/WBSITE/EXTERNAL/PROJECTS/0,,menuPK:115635~pagePK:64020917~piPK:64021009~theSitePK:40941,00.html.

[73] Global Fund, http://www.theglobalfund.org/en/about/how/.

[74] Global Fund, http://www.theglobalfund.org/en/funds_raised/commitments/.

- Grant commitments represent liabilities based on signed grant agreements or in the case of those countries with pending grant agreements (not yet signed), the dollar value of a proposal approved by the Global Fund board.
- Disbursements represent actual payments made by the Global Fund to grant recipients.

The database can be searched by region, country, funding round, two-year amount, and disease. Information about the funding amount and the text of the full grant proposal is also available.

List of Interviewees

Interviewee	Affiliation	Title
Julia Benn	OECD/DAC (Organisation for Economic Co-operation and Development/Development Assistance Committee)	Administrator, Statistics and Monitoring Division, Development Co-operation Directorate (DCD)
Stan Bernstein	Millennium Project (formerly from UNFPA)	Sexual and Reproductive Health Policy Adviser
Susna De	PHR*plus* (Partners for Health Reform*plus*)/Abt Associates	Coordinator, PHR*plus* National Health Accounts Initiative
Paul De Lay	UNAIDS (Joint United Nations Programme on HIV/AIDS)	Director, Monitoring and Evaluation
Tania Dmytraczenko	PHR*plus*/Abt Associates	Health Economist and Associate
Jacqueline Eckhardt-Gerritson	NIDI (Netherlands Interdisciplinary Demographic Institute)	Project Leader, Resource Flows Project
Sarah Ewart	Malaria Vaccine Initiative	Policy Analyst
Katherine Floyd	WHO (World Health Organization)	Stop TB Department
Charo Garg	WHO	Health Economist, Health System Financing, Expenditure & Resource Allocation
Brian Hammond	OECD/DAC	Head, Statistics and Monitoring Division, DCD
Jose-Antonio Izazola–Licea	SIDALAC (Regional AIDS Initiative for Latin America & Caribbean)	Executive Coordinator
Kei Kawabata	WHO	Coordinator of Resource Flows, Expenditures, and Risk Protection Team
Patience Kuruneri	WHO	Senior Adviser, Roll Back Malaria Partnership Secretariat
Eric Lief	Independent consultant	Former Senior Advisory Resource Coordination, UNAIDS
Patrick Lydon	WHO	Health Economist, Immunization, Vaccines, and Biologicals Department
Bill McGreevey	The Futures Group International	Director, Development Economics
Catherine Michaud	Harvard Center for Population and Development Studies	Senior Research Associate
Paul Nunn	WHO	Coordinator, TB/HIV and Drug Resistance, Stop TB Department
Ann Pawlicsko	UNFPA (United Nations Populations Fund)	NIDI Monitor
Lisa Regis	UNAIDS	
Barbara Seligman	USAID (U.S. Agency for International Development)	Senior Policy Advisor, Bureau of Global Health
Ruben Suarez-Berenguela	National Health Accounts, Pan American Health Organization (PAHO)	Economic Advisor, EquiLAC

Interview Questions About Health Resource Tracking

Questions About Resource Tracking of Health Related Monies, Goods, and Services

1. What is the main mission of your organization? Is resource tracking of health resources part of that mission?
2. Why are you tracking health resources?
3. For which health needs/diseases are you tracking the provision of resources? AIDS, TB, malaria, childhood vaccinations, other health care related needs?
4. For which countries are you tracking health resources?
5. What types of health related resources are you tracking? Monetary? In-kind goods and services?
6. What types of information are you collecting? Funds committed or disbursed for health care purposes? In-country use of funds received?
7. From whom do you collect this information? (governments, NGOs, foundations, etc.)
8. How do you collect this information? (interviews, surveys, etc.) May we have a copy of what you use?
9. How current is the information that you collect? How often do you collect this information?
10. When did you start tracking/collecting information on health resources? How many years do you have information for?
11. How detailed is the information? (e.g., Are the data aggregated or detailed? Are the data detailed enough that individual donations can be tracked?)
12. Who uses this information?
13. For what is the information used? (e.g., policymaking; project monitoring and evaluation; assessing public health needs; conducting infectious disease surveillance; allocating health care resources; determining the true costs of specific types of health care; eliminating errors in and improving the overall quality of health care)
14. What information is available to the public?
15. What additional information would you like to collect/track if it were available/possible (i.e., what gaps exist)?
16. Have you identified any other gaps in the collection or reporting of health care resources?
17. Who else is tracking similar information that you think we should talk to?

References

Abel-Smith, B., "Paying for Health Services: A Study of Costs and Sources of Finance in Six Countries," Geneva: World Health Organization, Public Health Papers No. 17, 1963.

Abel-Smith, B., "An International Study of Health Expenditure and Its Relevance for Health," Geneva: World Health Organization, Public Health Papers No. 32, 1967.

Commission of the European Communities, International Monetary Fund, Organisation for Economic Co-operation and Development, United Nations, and World Bank, *System of National Accounts 1993*, Brussels/Luxembourg, New York, Paris, Washington, D.C., 1993. Available at http://unstats.un.org/unsd/sna1993/toctop.asp.

Davey, M. E., and R. E. Rowberg, "Challenges in Collecting and Reporting Federal Research and Development Data," Congressional Research Service Report to Congress, January 31, 2000.

Funders Concerned About AIDS, *Report on HIV-AIDS Grantmaking by U.S. Philanthropy, November 2003,* New York: FCAA, 2003.

Guthrie, T., and A. Hickey (eds.), *Funding the Fight: Budgeting for HIV/AIDS in Developing Countries*, Cape Town: Idasa AIDS Budget Unit, October 2004.

Hickey, A., N. Ndlovu, and T. Guthrie, *Budgeting for HIV/AIDS in South Africa: Report on Intergovernmental Funding Flows for an Integrated Response in the Social Sector,* Cape Town: Idasa Budget Information Service, 2003.

Hjortsberg, C., "Issue Paper on National Health Accounts—Where Are We Today?" Swedish International Development Cooperation Agency (SIDA) Health Division, Document 2001:6, 2001.

Joint United Nations Programme on HIV/AIDS, *Country Response Information System: Overview of the System and Its Plan of Establishment*, Geneva: UNAIDS, 2003.

Kates, J., and T. Summers, "U.S. Government Funding for Global HIV/AIDS Through FY 2005," Kaiser Family Foundation, Policy Brief, December 2004.

Ndlovu, N., "Where Is HIV/AIDS in the Budget? Survey of 2002 Provincial Social Sector Budgets," Cape Town: Idasa Budget Information Service, 2003.

Organisation for Economic Co-operation and Development, *A System of Health Accounts*, Paris: OECD, 2000.

Organisation for Economic Co-operation and Development, *OECD Health Data 2004: A Comparative Analysis of 30 Countries—User's Guide.* Paris: OECD, 2004. Available at http://www.oecd.org/document/51/0,2340,en_2649_34631_2085235_1_1_1_1,00.html.

Pan American Health Organization, *Health Conditions in the Americas, 1994 Edition, Volumes I and II,* Washington, D.C.: PAHO, 1994.

Pan American Health Organization, *Health in the Americas, 2002 Edition, Volumes I and II,* Washington, D.C.: PAHO, Scientific and Technical Publication No. 587, 2002.

Pan American Health Organization, "Health Accounts and National Health Accounts in the Americas, Executive Summary," Washington, D.C.: PAHO, 2003.

Pan American Health Organization and World Health Organization, *Data Base of Trade in Health Related Goods and Services in the Americas,* Washington, D.C.: PAHO, July 2003.

Partners for Health Reform*plus,* "Using NHA to Inform the Policy Process," Bethesda, MD: Partners for Health Reform*plus* Project, Abt Associates Inc., NHA Global Policy Brief, 2002.

Partners for Health Reform*plus, National Health Accounts Training Manual,* Bethesda, MD: Partners for Health Reform*plus* Project, Abt Associates Inc., 2003a.

Partners for Health Reform*plus, Primer for Policymakers—Understanding National Health Accounts: The Methodology and Implementation Process,* Bethesda, MD: Partners for Health Reform*plus* Project, Abt Associates Inc., May 2003b.

Rannan-Eliya, R., P. Berman, and A. Somanathan, *Health Accounting: A Comparison of the System of National Health Accounts and National Health Accounts Approaches,* Bethesda, MD: Partnerships for Health Reform Project, Abt Associates Inc., Special Initiative Report No. 4, December 1997.

Regional AIDS Initiative for Latin America and the Caribbean, *Technical Handbook for Estimating the National Health Accounts on HIV/AIDS: National Estimation of Financial Flows and Expenditures on HIV/AIDS,* Tepepan, Mexico: Fundación Mexicana para la Salud, A.C., 2001.

Summers, T., and J. Kates, "Global Funding for HIV/AIDS in Resource Poor Settings," Menlo Park: CA, Kaiser Family Foundation, Policy Brief 6051-02, December 2003a.

Summers T., and J. Kates, "U.S. Government Funding for HIV/AIDS in Resource Poor Settings," Menlo Park, CA: Kaiser Family Foundation, Issue Brief 6050-02, December 2003b.

United Nations, "Implementation of the United Nations Millennium Declaration: Report of the Secretary-General," New York: United Nations General Assembly, A/58/323, September 2, 2003. Available at http://ods-dds-ny.un.org/doc/UNDOC/GEN/N03/481/57/PDF/N0348157.pdf?OpenElement.

United Nations, "The Flow of Financial Resources for Assisting in the Implementation of the Programme of Action of the International Conference on Population and Development: A Ten-Year Review Report of the Secretary-General," New York: United Nations General Assembly, E/CN.9/2004/4, January 2004.

United Nations Development Programme, *Human Development Report 2003: Millennium Development Goals: A Compact Among Nations to End Human Poverty,* New York: UNDP, 2003.

United Nations Population Fund, *Global Population Assistance Report 1982–1988,* New York: UNFPA, 1989.

United Nations Population Fund, *Financial Resource Flows for Population Activities in 2002,* New York: UNFPA, 2004. Available at http://www.unfpa.org/publications/detail.cfm?ID=212&filterListType=

Webb, E. J., D. T. Campbell, R. D. Schwartz, and L. Sechrest, *Unobtrusive Measures: Nonreactive Research in the Social Sciences,* Chicago, IL: RAND McNally & Co., 1966.

World Bank, *World Development Indicators 2004*, Washington, D.C.: World Bank Group, 2004.

World Health Organization, *National Health Accounts: Concepts, Data Sources and Methodology*, Geneva: WHO, WHO/EIP/02.47, 2002.

World Health Organization, *The World Health Report 2003—Shaping the Future*, Geneva: WHO, 2003. Available at http://www.who.int/whr/previous/en/.

World Health Organization, *Global Tuberculosis Control: Surveillance, Planning, Financing*, Geneva: WHO, WHO/HTM/TB/2004.331, 2004a.

World Health Organization, *The World Health Report 2004—Changing History*, Geneva: WHO, 2004b. Available at http://www.who.int/whr/2004/en/.

World Health Organization, World Bank, and United States Agency for International Development, *Guide to Producing National Health Accounts: With Special Application to Low-Income and Middle-Income Countries*, Geneva: WHO, 2003.